Transforaminal Full-Endoscopic Lumbar Surgery Under the Local Anesthesia

Koichi Sairyo
Editor

Transforaminal Full-Endoscopic Lumbar Surgery Under the Local Anesthesia

State of the Art

Springer

Editor
Koichi Sairyo
Professor and Chairman
Department of Orthopedics
Tokushima University
Tokushima
Japan

ISBN 978-981-15-7022-3 ISBN 978-981-15-7023-0 (eBook)
https://doi.org/10.1007/978-981-15-7023-0

This Springer imprint is published by the registered company Springer Nature Singapore Pte Ltd.
The registered company address is: 152 Beach Road, #21-01/04 Gateway East, Singapore 189721, Singapore

I dedicate this book to my children, Eriko, Yuya, and Rena.
Their encouragement always drives my passion for creating new surgical technology.
To my wife, Michiko, thank you for your unending understanding of my challenge.

KOICHI SAIRYO

Preface

The purpose of this textbook is to provide a comprehensive overview of transforaminal (TF) full-endoscopic lumbar spine surgery (FESS) under local anesthesia. This technique started more than two decades ago, and it was introduced in Japan in 2003 by Professor Dezawa, my mentor. In the two decades, the endoscopic technique and equipment have evolved greatly and rapidly. However even now, we do not have appropriate textbooks on this technique in Japanese and in English.

I am a professor and chairman in the Department of Orthopedics at Tokushima University, Japan. I am the only professor in Japan who has been conducting TF-FESS. So far, I have instructed my technique to many fellows in my department. Thus, many surgeons have been doing full-endoscopic spine surgery in Tokushima University and affiliated hospitals. In Japan, Tokushima would be Mecca of TF-FESS, I hope. This textbook covers almost all areas of TF-FESS, including its history, anatomy, discectomy, decompression surgery, intradiscal therapy, fullendo KLIF surgery, and so on. The authors are all my fellows in Tokushima University. I am very glad that Tokushima University could make this outstanding textbook. I now decide that I should keep challenging to change the gold standard of spine surgery using TF-FESS.

Tokushima, Japan

Koichi Sairyo

Contents

Part I

Overview

History of Transforaminal Full-Endoscopic Lumbar Surgery

1

Koichi Sairyo and Toru Maeda

Abstract

Transforaminal approach was started as the technique of percutaneous discectomy by Hijikata in Japan. Hijikata's method was minimally invasive; however, it could not remove the entire herniated mass in the spinal canal because he did not use the endoscope. From the later 1980s, a trial was started by Kambin, Schreiber and Leu to utilize an endoscope or arthroscope in the percutaneous discectomy technique. The current single-portal endoscopic discectomy was established by Anthony Yeung. Initially, the indication was only for the herniated nucleus pulposus. Nowadays, thanks to the development of the instruments and high-speed drill, the indication enlarged to the spinal canal stenosis. These full-endoscopic spinal surgeries can be done under local anesthesia with 8 mm skin incision. This must be the least invasive spine surgery.

Keywords

Full-endoscopic spine surgery · Kambin triangle · Local anesthesia · Transforaminal approach

1.1 History of the Transforaminal Approach

Historically, the transforaminal full-endoscopic lumbar surgery would be based on the percutaneous technique of the discectomy by Hijikata [1, 2]. The benefit of the approach is that it is conducted under local anesthesia with minimal invasiveness. Kambin was another pioneer of this approach [3–5]. Figure 1.1 represents Kambin's triangle. The exiting nerve is the anterior aspect, and superior articular process is the

K. Sairyo (✉) · T. Maeda
Department of Orthopedics, Tokushima University, Tokushima, Japan

K. Sairyo (ed.), *Transforaminal Full-Endoscopic Lumbar Surgery Under the Local Anesthesia*, https://doi.org/10.1007/978-981-15-7023-0_1

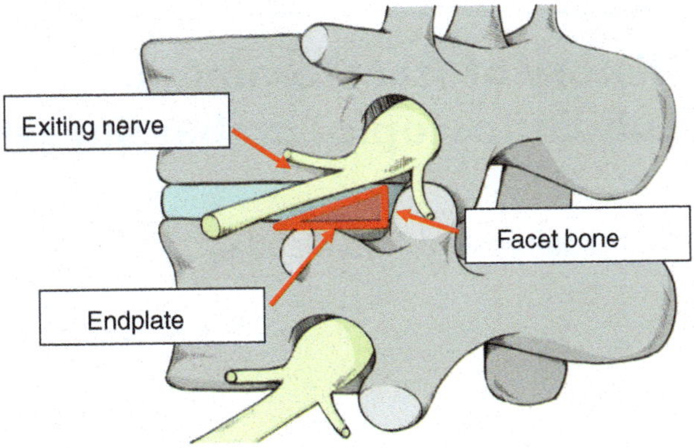

Fig. 1.1 Kambin triangle

medial aspect. The endplate of the caudal vertebral body is the inferior aspect of the triangle. As for the percutaneous discectomy technique, a cannula is inserted through the Kambin's triangle safely into the disc. However, without an endoscope, it was difficult to remove disc fragments located inside the canal. Thus, the trial to use the endoscope with the percutaneous discectomy was initiated.

1.2 History of the Transforaminal Endoscopic Technique

From the later 1980s, a trial was started by Kambin, Schreiber and Leu to utilize an endoscope or arthroscope in the percutaneous discectomy technique [6, 7]. The current single-portal endoscopic discectomy was established by Anthony Yeung et al. [8–10]. The use of a spinal endoscope improves reliability when removing an HNP compared with Hijikata's conventional technique. Initially, they named the technique [11] as selective endoscopic discectomy (SED).

Recently, Dezawa [12, 13] further established an advanced technique using a high-speed drill which enables most HNPs to be removed. In Asia, they call the technique as percutaneous endoscopic discectomy (PED). On the other hand, in Europe [14–16] a similar technique is called full-endoscopic discectomy (FED). In different regions of the world, different terms are used such as SED, PED, or FED. In 2018, regional representatives from all over the world discussed on its nomenclature. Finally, they reached a consensus in favor of the name of the procedure as full-endoscopic surgery, not selected or percutaneous endoscopic technique [17]. Afterwards in Asia including our country Japan, we decided to use full-endoscopic not percutaneous technique.

1.3 History of the Development of the Surgical Indication

Transforaminal (TF) full-endoscopic surgery was first indicated for lumbar discectomy (FELD). It requires only 8 mm skin incision, and muscle damage is minimum. Moreover, it can be done under local anesthesia. The TF-FELD must be the minimally invasive spine surgery, currently. At the beginning, the disc fragment around

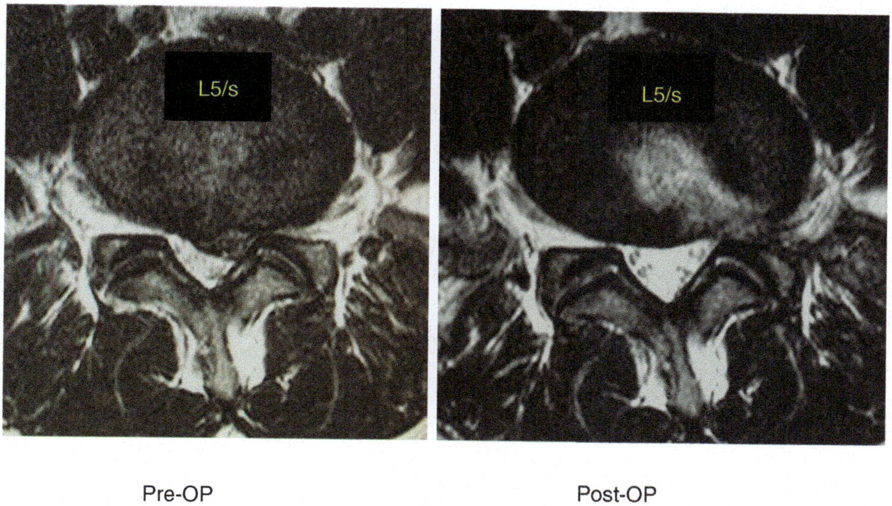

Fig. 1.2 MRIs before and after the TF-FELD at L5/s

the disc space was in the good indication. After a specially made high-speed drill for the FED system was invented [13, 18, 19], the indication is enlarged. By using the high speed drill, foraminotomy and partial pediculotomy are possible, so that the foraminal space gets bigger. In such bigger working foraminal space [19], the cannula can be inserted intracanalicular space at the L5/s level. Figure 1.2 demonstrates MRIs before and after the TF-FELD at L5/s. Also, after foraminoplasty, outside-in surgery can be safely done [20].

The next step is the application for lumbar spinal canal stenosis. The majority of patients with spinal canal stenosis is elderly people. The TF approach is possible with local anesthesia; thus, it should greatly benefit those, especially the elderly cases, with poor general condition. First, the foraminal stenosis was decompressed with TF full-endoscopic system [21, 22]. Now, it is called transforaminal endoscopic lumbar foraminotomy (TELF) or TF-FELF (full-endoscopic lumbar foraminotomy). Figure 1.3 demonstrates CTs before and after the TF-FELF. The gold standard surgery for foraminal stenosis would be spinal fusion after the facetectomy. Thus, TF-FELF under local anesthesia must be by far the one that has great benefits for the elderly cases.

Second, lateral recess stenosis can be decompressed with the TF approach [23–26]. We called the technique as TF-FEVF (full-endoscopic ventral facetectomy), since the decompressed area is the ventral aspect of the facet joint. In the consensus paper [17], it is called as TE-LRD (transforaminal full-endoscopic lateral recess decompression). The lateral recess decompression would be easier using the interlaminar approach. However, interlaminar approach requires general anesthesia. The TF-FEVF is possible under local anesthesia. This would greatly benefit the elderly cases with poor general condition such as poor pulmonary or cardiac condition. Figure 1.4 demonstrates CTs before and after the TF-FEVF at L4/5. It is clear that the lateral recess is decompressed.

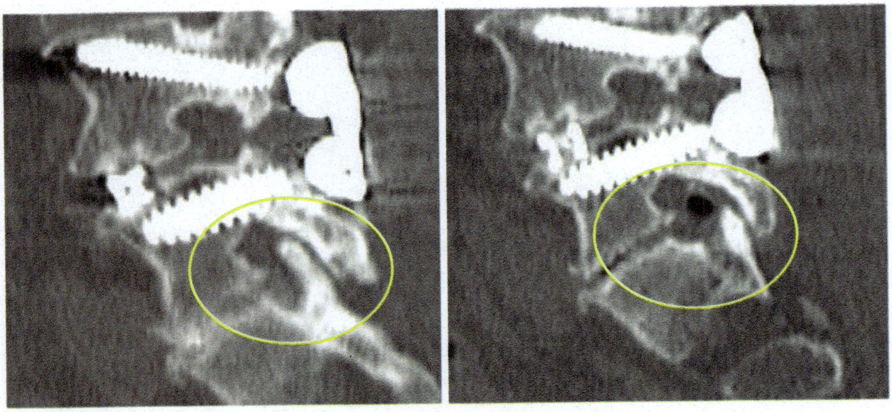

Pre-OP Post-OP

Fig. 1.3 CTs before and after the TF-FELF at L5/s

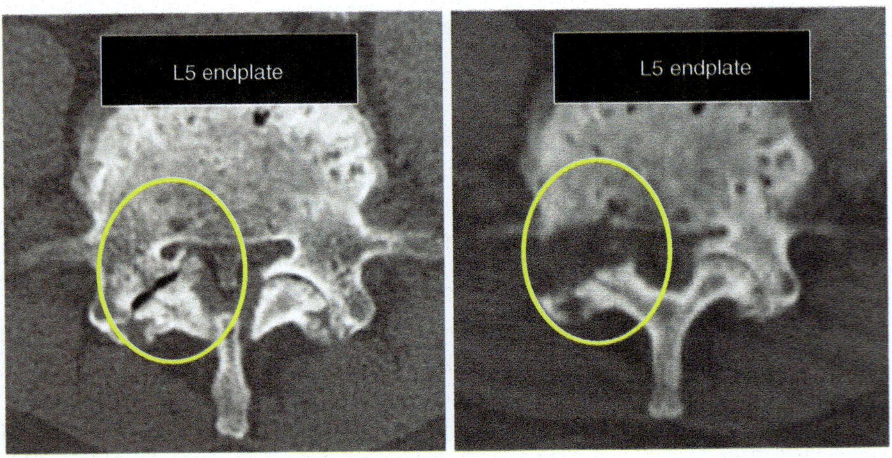

Pre-OP Post-OP

Fig. 1.4 CTs before and after the TF-FEVF at L4/5

References

1. Hijikata S. A method of percutaneous nuclear extraction. J Toden Hosp. 1975;5:39.
2. Hijikata S. Percutaneous nucleotomy. A new concept technique and 12 years' experience. Clin Orthop Relat Res. 1989;238:9–23.
3. Kambin P, Sampson S. Posterolateral percutaneous suction-excision of herniated lumbar intervertebral discs. Report of interim results. Clin Orthop Relat Res. 1986;207:37–43.
4. Kambin P, Brager MD. Percutaneous posterolateral discectomy. Anatomy and mechanism. Clin Orthop Relat Res. 1987;223:145–54.
5. Kambin P, Schaffer JL. Percutaneous lumbar discectomy. Review of 100 patients and current practice. Clin Orthop Relat Res. 1989;238:24–34.

6. Kambin P. Arthroscopic microdiskectomy. Mt Sinai J Med. 1991;58(2):159–64.
7. Schreiber A, Leu H. Percutaneous nucleotomy: technique with discoscopy. Orthopedics. 1991;14(4):439–44.
8. Yeung AT. The evolution of percutaneous spinal endoscopy and discectomy: state of the art. Mt Sinai J Med. 2000;67:327–32.
9. Yeung AT, Tsou PM. Posterolateral endoscopic excision for lumbar disc herniation: surgical technique, outcome, and complications in 307 consecutive cases. Spine. 2002;27:722–31.
10. Yeung AT, Yeung CA. Minimally invasive techniques for the management of lumbar disc herniation. Orthop Clin North Am. 2007;38(3):363–72.
11. Tsou PM, Alan Yeung C, Yeung AT. Posterolateral transforaminal selective endoscopic discectomy and thermal annuloplasty for chronic lumbar discogenic pain: a minimal access visualized intradiscal surgical procedure. Spine J. 2004;4(5):564–73.
12. Dezawa A, Sairyo K. New minimally invasive discectomy technique through the interlaminar space using a percutaneous endoscope. Asian J Endosc Surg. 2011;4(2):94–8.
13. Dezawa A, Mikami H, Sairyo K. Percutaneous endoscopic translaminar approach for herniated nucleus pulposus in the hidden zone of the lumbar spine. Asian J Endosc Surg. 2012;5(4):200–3.
14. Ruetten S, Komp M, Merk H, Godolias G. Use of newly developed instruments and endoscopes: full-endoscopic resection of lumbar disc herniations via the interlaminar and lateral transforaminal approach. J Neurosurg Spine. 2007;6(6):521–30.
15. Ruetten S, Komp M, Merk H, Godolias G. Full-endoscopic interlaminar and transforaminal lumbar discectomy versus conventional microsurgical technique: a prospective, randomized, controlled study. Spine (Phila Pa 1976). 2008;33(9):931–9.
16. Birkenmaier C, Komp M, Leu HF, Wegener B, Ruetten S. The current state of endoscopic disc surgery: review of controlled studies comparing full-endoscopic procedures for disc herniations to standard procedures. Pain Physician. 2013;16(4):335–44.
17. Hofstetter CP, Choi G, Gibson JNA, Ruetten S, Zhou Y, Wagner R, Ahn Y, Lee JH, Sairyo K, Telfeian AE, Prada N, Shen J, Cortinas FC, Brooks NP, Van Daele P, Kotheeranurak V, Hasan S, Härtl R, Kim JS. AO consensus paper on nomenclature for working channel endoscopic spinal procedures. Global Spine J. 2020;10(2 Suppl):111S–121S. https://doi.org/10.1177/2192568219887364. Epub 2020 May 28.
18. Henmi T, Terai T, Hibino N, Yoshioka S, Kondo K, Goda Y, Tezuka F, Sairyo K. Percutaneous endoscopic lumbar discectomy utilizing ventral epiduroscopic observation technique and foraminoplasty for transligamentous extruded nucleus pulposus: technical note. J Neurosurg Spine. 2016;24(2):275–80.
19. Henmi T, Terai T, Nagamachi A, Sairyo K. Morphometric changes of the lumbar intervertebral foramen after percutaneous endoscopic foraminoplasty under local anesthesia. J Neurol Surg A Cent Eur Neurosurg. 2018;79(1):19–24.
20. Yoshinari H, Tezuka F, Yamashita K, Manabe H, Hayashi F, Ishihama Y, Sugiura K, Takata Y, Sakai T, Maeda T, Sairyo K. Transforaminal full-endoscopic lumbar discectomy under local anesthesia in awake and aware conditions: the inside-out and outside-in techniques. Curr Rev Musculoskelet Med. 2019;12:311–7.
21. Yamashita K, Higashino K, Sakai T, Takata Y, Hayashi F, Tezuka F, Morimoto M, Chikawa T, Nagamachi A, Sairyo K. Percutaneous full endoscopic lumbar foraminoplasty for adjacent level foraminalstenosis following vertebral intersegmental fusion in an awake and aware patient under local anesthesia: a case report. J Med Invest. 2017;64(3.4):291–5.
22. Yeung A, Gore S. Endoscopic foraminal decompression for failed back surgery syndrome under local anesthesia. Int J Spine Surg. 2014;8 https://doi.org/10.14444/1022. eCollection 2014.
23. Sairyo K, Higashino K, Yamashita K, Hayashi F, Wada K, Sakai T, Takata Y, Tezuka F, Morimoto M, Terai T, Chikawa T, Yonezu H, Nagamachi A, Fukui Y. A new concept of transforaminal ventral facetectomy including simultaneous decompression of foraminal and lateral recess stenosis: technical considerations in a fresh cadaver model and a literature review. J Med Invest. 2017;64(1.2):1–6.

24. Lewandrowski KU. Endoscopic transforaminal and lateral recess decompression after previous spinal surgery. Int J Spine Surg. 2018;12(2):98–111.
25. Nakajima D, Yamashita K, Tezuka F, Manabe H, Ishihama Y, Sugiura K, Takata Y, Sakai T, Maeda T, Sairyo K. Successful percutaneous endoscopic decompression surgery under the local anesthesia for L5 radiculopathy caused by L5-S1 foraminal stenosis and L4-5 lateral recess stenosis: a case report. J Med Investig. 2020;67(1.2):192–6.
26. Sugiura K, Yamashita K, Manabe H, Ishihama Y, Tezuka F, Takata Y, Sakai T, Maeda T, Sairyo K. Prompt return to work after bilateral transforaminal full-endoscopic lateral recess decompression under local anesthesia: a case report. J Neurol Surg A. 2020. in press.

Anatomy for Full Endoscopic Discectomy (FED) via Transforaminal Approach

2

Kosaku Higashino, Hiroaki Manabe, Yasuaki Tamaki, Nori Sato, Tomohiro Goto, Koichi Tomita, Yoshihiro Tsuruo, and Koichi Sairyo

Abstract

For normal surgery, it is recommended that surgeons approach the operative field without developing a critical site. Especially, minimally invasive surgery sometimes only requires anatomical knowledge at the trajectory field because understanding further confirmation of a surrounding tissue or an organ is difficult.

For surgeons, lack of opportunity to learn the field outside the surgery site may cause a stumbling block in the progress of the procedure. It is useful for the continued progress of reliable and safe minimally invasive surgery to understand the distribution of the circumference of the organ and the tissue. The Kambin's triangle approach is the conventional safe transforaminal approach (Kambin and Brager, Clin Orthop Relat Res (223):145–154, 1987). However, the safe triangle approach sometimes may cause irritation of the spinal nerve root because of severe spinal stenosis, epidural fibrosis, and intervertebral disk degeneration.

We report anatomical findings necessary for full-endoscopic discectomy (FED) via the transforaminal approach.

Keywords

Anatomy · Lumbar plexus · Posterior ramus of spinal nerve · Ligamentum flavum

K. Higashino (✉)
Department of Orthopedics, Sikoku Medical Center for Children and Adults, Zentsuji City, Kagawa, Japan

H. Manabe · Y. Tamaki · N. Sato · T. Goto · K. Sairyo
Department of Orthopedics, Tokushima University, Tokushima, Japan

K. Tomita · Y. Tsuruo
Department of Anatomy, Tokushima University, Tokushima, Japan

K. Sairyo (ed.), *Transforaminal Full-Endoscopic Lumbar Surgery Under the Local Anesthesia*, https://doi.org/10.1007/978-981-15-7023-0_2

2.1 Introduction

For normal surgery, it is recommended that we approach it without developing a critical site. Observing the site by clinical dissection allows opening the operative approach. For normal surgery, it is recommended that we approach it without developing a critical site. Observing the site by clinical dissection allows opening the operative approach. For surgeons, lack of opportunity to learn the field outside the surgery site may cause a stumbling block in the progress of the procedure. It is useful for the continued progress of reliable and safe minimally invasive surgery to understand the distribution of the circumference of the organ and the tissue. The Kambin's triangle approach is the conventional safe transforaminal approach [1]. However, the safe triangle approach sometimes may cause irritation of the spinal nerve root because of severe spinal stenosis, epidural fibrosis, and intervertebral disk degeneration.

We have experienced an opportunity to review other operative fields at a time aside from the systematic anatomical dissection and to being alerted to the true findings. For the lumbar plexus, only the main nerves are explained in the dissection; however, we can confirm the network of many nerve fibers through systemic dissection [2, 3].

Also, the ligamentum flavum does not attach from top to bottom across the vertebrae uniformly, and it is found be thicker in the dorsum of the lumbar vertebrae and to cover the joint [4–6]. Because it is difficult in this report to introduce the dissection of the entire backbone and the spinal cord, we report only lumbar vertebrae nerves, the posterior longitudinal ligament, the lumbar disc, and the ligamentum flavum using a lumbar specimen.

2.2 Lumbar Plexus

The lumbar plexus in an atlas introduced when the psoas major muscle is resected to simplify the main nerves. However, when local dissection is actually performed using the lumbar specimen with resected psoas major muscle, the lumbar plexus was shown to have innumerable nerve fiber networks in the psoas muscle, and it may be not consistent among individuals (Fig. 2.1) [2, 3]. Dissection raises the risk of nerve injury if insertion is from outside the safety triangle via the transforaminal approach. In the case of stimulating an exiting nerve root during surgery via the transforaminal approach, this is the point where you should be careful about changing the insertion trajectory.

2.3 Foramen Ligament

Many authors report anatomical findings about the foramen ligament. The ligamentous distribution varies according to the individual lumbar vertebral level [7–9]. The foramen ligament is distributed in a form to cover the foramen

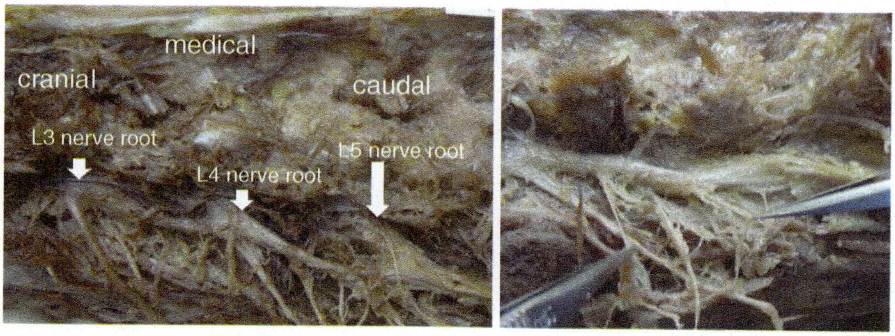

Fig. 2.1 Lumbar plexus from L3 to L5 levels shows innumerable nerve fibers made of a network form

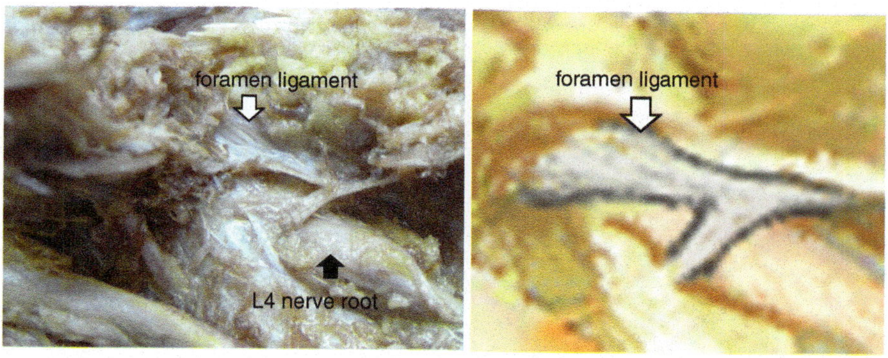

Fig. 2.2 Foramen ligament at left L4–L5 is distributed in a form to cover the foramen

(Fig. 2.2). These ligaments have a role in the stability of each lumbar nerve root; however, these ligaments can cause a decrease in the range of motion of the nerve root [8].

2.4 Dorsal Ramus of the Lumbar Nerve

The dorsal ramus of the lumbar nerve is divided into a medial branch and a lateral branch [2]. The articular branch at the facet joint branches off from the medial branch, and blood vessels accompany the medial branch (Fig. 2.3). The dissection view showed that another medial branch from the lower nerve root is distributed on the facet joint. Superior or inferior nerve branches are distributed through the foraminal area, which surgeons should note.

This report depends on the details in the literature. Nerve terminals to the intervertebral joint dorsum are also reported [2, 3, 10].

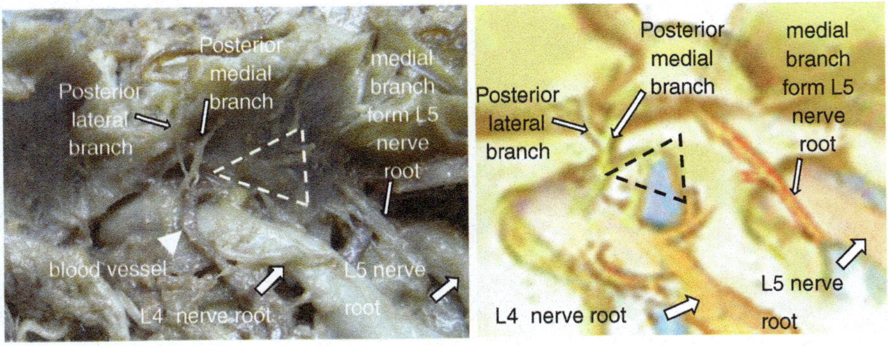

Fig. 2.3 Articular branch from the nerve root shown at left L4–L5 facet joint. One medial branch is distributed from L5 nerve root and a blood vessel accompanied the medial branch from L4 nerve root. *White and black dots triangle* show safe triangle area

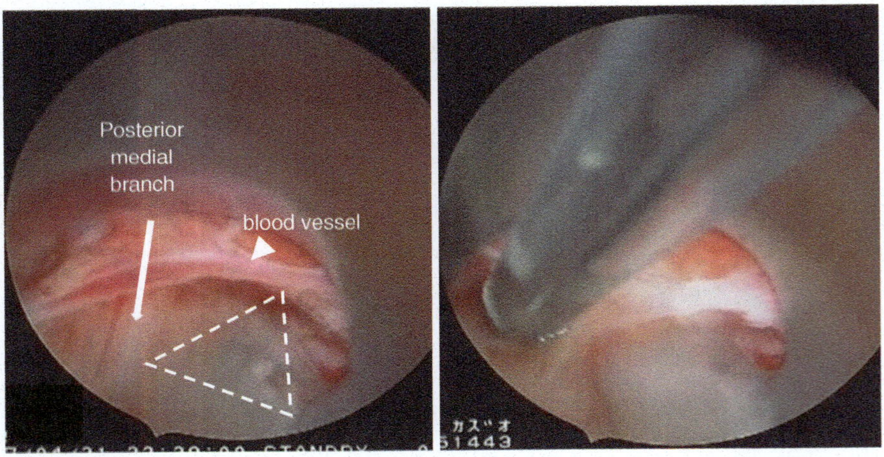

Fig. 2.4 Articular branch from nerve root (*white arrow*) shown at left L4–L5 facet joint. Blood vessel accompanies medial branch (*white arrowhead*). *White dots triangle* shows safe triangle. In bipolar coagulation, the patient felt pain in the innervation area (*right panel*)

2.5 Anatomy for Lumbar Disc at Posterior Lesion: The Posterior Longitudinal Ligament and Nerve Distribution

Study is taken up with intervertebral disc-related low back pain in the orthopedics region; however, the clinical condition of intervertebral disc-related low back pain is still unclear.

The posterior longitudinal ligament covers only the center of the dorsum of the vertebral body and spreads as a cross at the intervertebral disc caudal side (Fig. 2.4) [11].

Also, here it is inferred that there is a nerve fiber distributed directly from the dorsal root ganglion, and the lumbar vertebral intervertebral disc dorsum is closely associated with intervertebral disc-related low back pain [10].

2.6 Ligamentum Flavum

The ligamentum flavum is a ligament named by its color; the yellow depends on elastin. It is an elastic fiber, and the elastin compares it with other ligaments with elasticity [12].

However, elasticity is lost by aging, causing lumbar spinal canal stenosis. Figure 2.5 shows a lumbar specimen cut at the pedicle, with the dorsum observed from the ventral aspect. The ligamentum flavum of this specimen at L4–L5 is present in the caudal foramen area, and the ligamentum flavum is spread over the facet joint border (Fig. 2.6) [6]. The lateral margin of the ligamentum flavum is described as extending to the foramen with variations [4–6].

In the case of foraminoplasty, the ligamentum flavum may be exposed during drilling at the ventral site of the superior articular process.

Any level switches over from the dorsum to the joint capsule of the intervertebral joint when we observe it, and it is inferred that we contribute to the stability of the intervertebral joint (Fig. 2.6) [4, 13, 14].

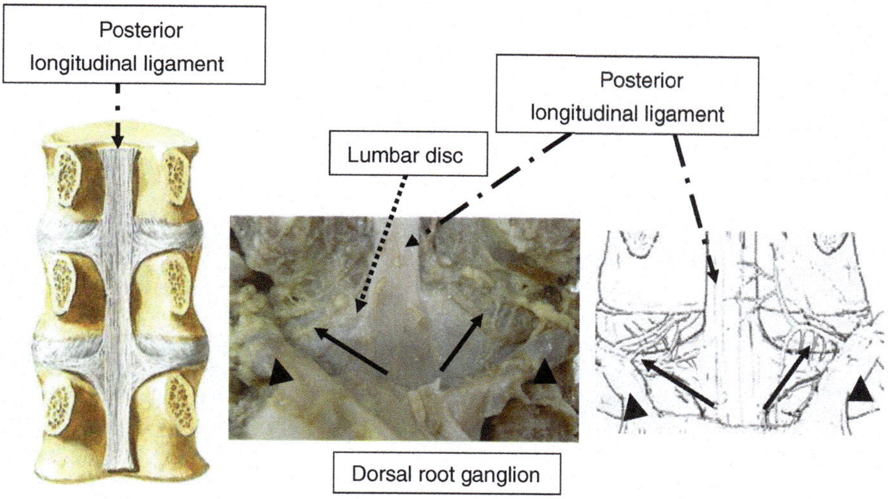

Fig. 2.5 Dura mater reversed to caudal side. Posterior longitudinal ligament is distributed over ten characters. Innervation to a backward intervertebral disc is distributed from dorsal root ganglion directly and thickly

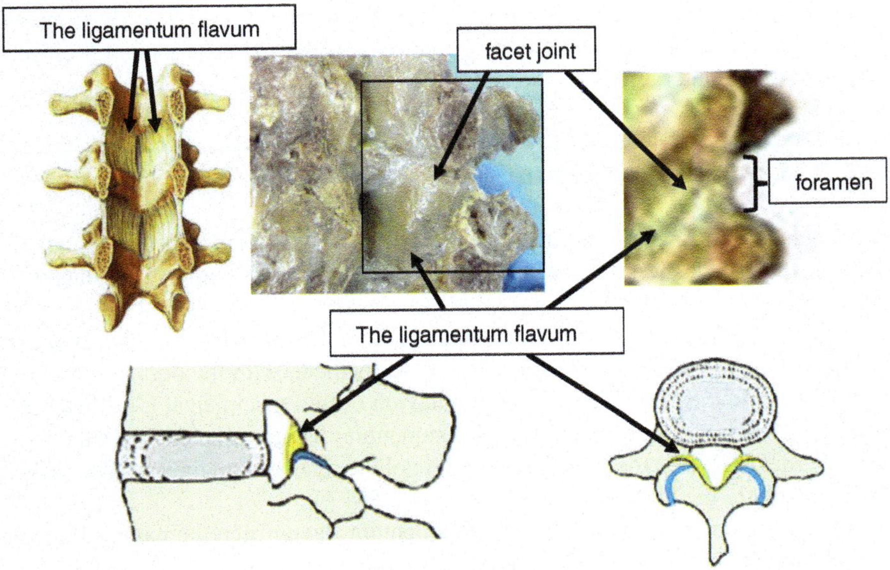

Fig. 2.6 Ligamentum flavum of this specimen at L4–L5 is present in caudal foramen area. Ligamentum flavum is spread over facet joint border

2.7 Summary

We report an anatomical finding necessary for full endoscopic discectomy (FED) via the transforaminal approach. It is important that any surgeon review the anatomical findings.

References

1. Kambin P, Brager MD. Percutaneous posterolateral discectomy. Anatomy and mechanism. Clin Orthop Relat Res. 1987;(223):145–54.
2. Bogduk N. A reappraisal of the anatomy of the human lumbar erector spinae. J Anat. 1980;131(pt 3):525–40.
3. Bogduk N, Long DM. The anatomy of the so-called "articular nerves" and their relationship to facet denervation in the treatment of low-back pain. J Neurosurg. 1979;51(2):172–7.
4. Olszewski AD, Yaszemski MJ, White AA 3rd. The anatomy of the human lumbar ligamentum flavum. New observations and their surgical importance. Spine (Phila 1976). 1996;21(20):2307–12.
5. Zarzur E. Anatomic studies of the human ligamentum flavum. Anesth Analg. 1984;63(5):499–502.
6. Chau AM, Pelzer NR, Hampton J, Smith A, Seex KA, Stewart F, et al. Lateral extent and ventral laminar attachments of the lumbar ligamentum flavum: cadaveric study. Spine J. 2014;14(10):2467–71.
7. Caglar YY, Dolgun H, Ugur HC, Kahilogullari G, Tekdemir I, Elhan A. A ligament in the lumbar foramina: inverted Y ligament: an anatomic report. Spine (Phila 1976). 2004;29(14):1504–7.

8. Kraan GA, Smit TH, Hoogland PV, Snijders CJ. Lumbar extraforaminal ligaments act as a traction relief and prevent spinal nerve compression. Clin Biomech (Bristol). 2010;25(1):10–5.
9. Zhong E, Zhao Q, Shi B, Xie Y, Ding Z, Lv H, et al. The morphology and possible clinical significance of the intraforaminal ligaments in the entrance zones of the L1–L5 levels. Pain Physician. 2018;21(2):E157–65.
10. Bogduk N, Tynan W, Wilson AS. The nerve supply to the human lumbar intervertebral discs. J Anat. 1981;132(pt 1):39–56.
11. Adams MA, Hutton WC. The effect of posture on the lumbar spine. J Bone Joint Surg Br. 1985;67(4):625–9.
12. Sato N, Taniguchi T, Goda Y, Kosaka H, Higashino K, Sakai T, et al. Proteomic analysis of human tendon and ligament: solubilization and analysis of insoluble extracellular matrix in connective tissues. J Proteome Res. 2016;15(12):4709–21.
13. Pintar FA, Yoganandan N, Myers T, Elhagediab A, Sances A Jr. Biomechanical properties of human lumbar spine ligaments. J Biomech. 1992;25(11):1351–6.
14. Panjabi MM, White AA 3rd. Basic biomechanics of the spine. Neurosurgery. 1980;7(1):76–93.

3 Standard Procedure of the Transforaminal Approach and How to Perform Local Anesthesia (Inside-Out Method)

Toshinori Sakai

Abstract

The standard procedure of the transforaminal approach (inside-out method) and how to perform local anesthesia are presented in this chapter. Currently, several additional techniques such as "foraminoplasty" have been developed, and readers should refer to other chapters on those new additional techniques. In this chapter, several specific techniques and technical terms on this surgical procedure are introduced for readers' understanding. The most important thing is to avoid any complications during all steps.

Keywords

Full-endoscopic discectomy (FED) · Local anesthesia · Transforaminal approach

3.1 Preoperative Information

3.1.1 Surgical Indications and Contraindications for the Transforaminal Approach Under Local Anesthesia

Primarily, patients with lumbar intervertebral herniation (LDH) above L4–5 level are indicated for the transforaminal approach. For L5-S LDH, the iliac crest frequently intercepts insertion of the endoscope, and special techniques such as foraminoplasty are required when it is absolutely necessary to be performed. However, the location and size of the iliac crest have individual differences, and there are cases incapable of L4–5 LDH or feasible for L5-S LDH without any special techniques.

T. Sakai (✉)
Department of Orthopedics, Institute of Biomedical Sciences, Tokushima University Graduate School, Tokushima, Japan

K. Sairyo (ed.), *Transforaminal Full-Endoscopic Lumbar Surgery Under the Local Anesthesia*, https://doi.org/10.1007/978-981-15-7023-0_3

There is no contraindication by the type/location of LDH, but because migrated/sequestrated types are required for the advanced technique, those types are not recommended for beginners. In addition, the cases accompanied with apophyseal ring fracture are not indicated. Patients who are allergic to anesthetic drugs such as lidocaine are absolutely contraindicated. Also, patients who do not constitutionally and/or mentally fit for the surgery under local anesthesia and younger patients such as elementary school children are preferable to avoid though they are not contraindicated.

In our institution, discography is necessarily conducted under prone position, which is simulating the actual operative position, to confirm the feasibility of this surgery under local anesthesia as a preoperative test. If the patient cannot stand this examination, FED under local anesthesia is not feasible.

3.2 Standard Procedure of the Transforaminal Approach

3.2.1 How to Decide the Insertion Point

Firstly, we locate the insertion point at 8–12 cm laterally from the center of the patient's back of the affected intervertebral disc level. For the patient having large built physique, it can be 12–14 cm laterally. Our method on how to decide it is presented below.

3.2.1.1 Consideration for the Abdominal Organs and the Iliac Crest

To reach the affected intervertebral disc at higher spinal level as L1–2, L2–3 via transforaminal approach, as T12 rib or kidney is frequently located on the trajectory, it is advisable that the surgeon should start by a slightly smaller angle of insertion and gradually increase the angle using the hand-down technique. Conversely, to reach the intervertebral disc at lower spinal level as L4–5, L5-S, the iliac crest obstructs the trajectory. Preoperative surgical plan using MRI/CT scan is mandatory to avoid surgical complications.

3.2.1.2 Consideration for the Patient's Physique and the Soft Tissue Volume

Basically, the insertion point is determined according to the preoperative CT discography (CTD). In our institution, preoperative CTD is taken in prone position assuming actual surgery.

3.2.2 How to Perform Local Anesthesia

Basically, 1% lidocaine is used for local anesthesia, whose reference maximum dose is 200 mg for an adult patient. Three syringes (10, 5, 1 ml with lock function) are prepared. The 10 and 1 ml syringes are filled with 1% lidocaine, and the 5 ml

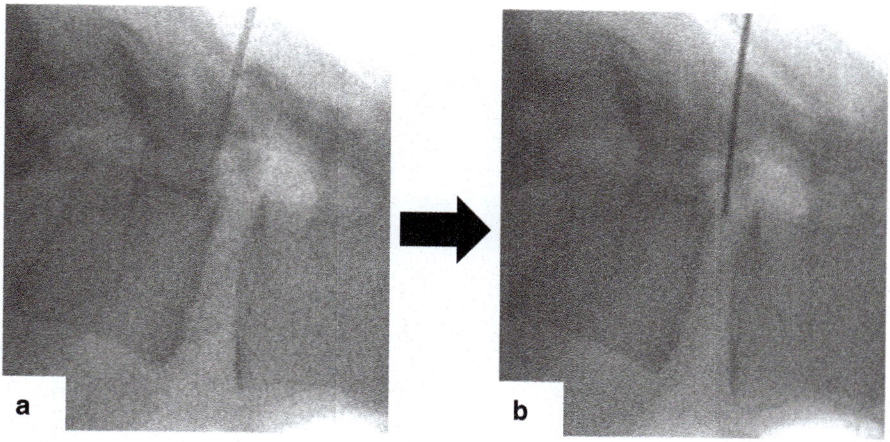

Fig. 3.1 If we directly insert a needle into the intervertebral disc, it frequently hits the exiting nerve root or sometimes goes into the epidural space through the foramen. Accordingly, at first, we place the needle at the superolateral wall of the pedicle of the vertebral body caudal to the target disc for safety (**a**). Next, the needle tip gradually moves caudally to the mid-lateral wall of the disc (**b**). This is called as "Waling technique"

syringe with the mixture composed of indigo carmine 2 ml, contrast medium 2 ml, and 1% lidocaine 1 ml.

After local anesthesia for the skin and subcutaneous tissue around the insertion point and trajectory with 1% lidocaine, next using the percutaneous transhepatic cholangial drainage (PTCD) needle, we place the needle at the superolateral wall of the pedicle of the vertebral body caudal to the affected (target) disc for safety. After local anesthesia around the pedicle with 1 ml of 1% lidocaine, the needle tip gradually moves caudally to the mid-lateral wall of the disc, which is called as the "Waling technique" (Fig. 3.1). In this step, if the needle tip touchs/stimulates the exiting nerve, the insertion point should be changed more medially. When the needle could be inserted 1 mm into the annulus fibrosus (AF) safely, whether the needle tip is located optimally should be confirmed by the A-P view (Fig. 3.2), and 1 ml of 1% lidocaine should be injected to the AF using the 1ml syringe with lock function. This location would be very important for this surgical procedure.

After the needle is set into the nucleus pulposus, the prepared mixture is injected gradually until the herniated mass is contrasted. Next, after the inner needle of the PTCD is removed, guide pin is inserted. Over the guide pin, the pencil-type obturator is inserted into the disc. Recently, to alleviate pain, we made a hole using the serial dilator.

3.2.3 How to Set the Endoscope

Over the pencil-type obturator, a cannula is set. There are three types of the cannula (straight type, duck bill type, oblique type) with the preference of a surgeon,

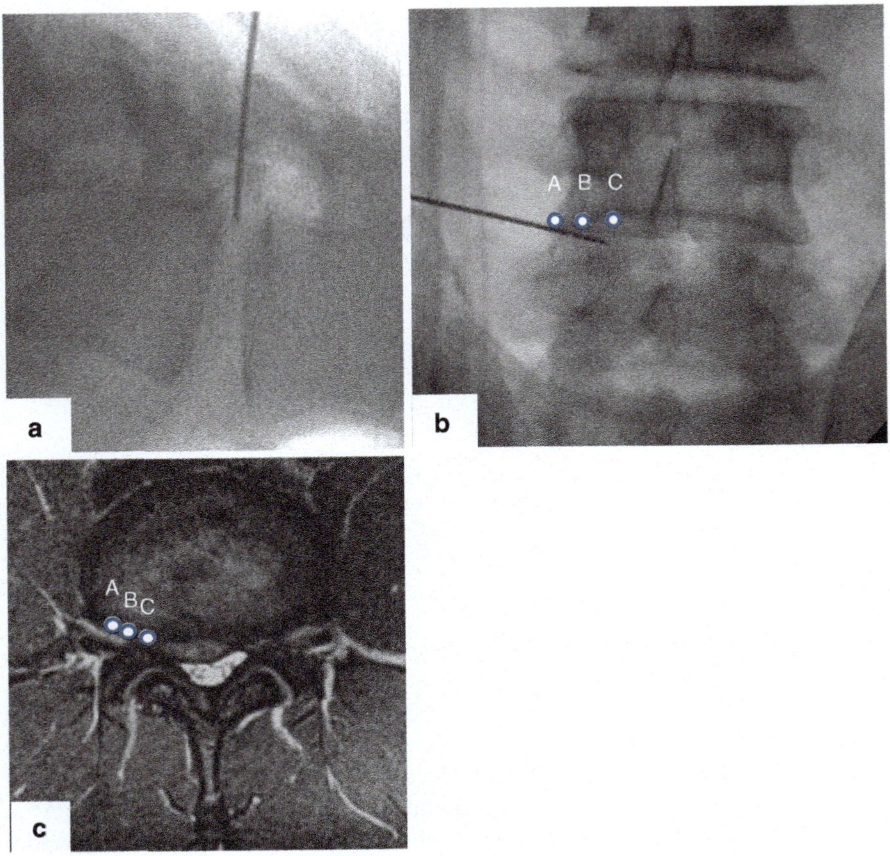

Fig. 3.2 When the needle could be inserted approximately 1 mm into the annulus fibrosus safely using lateral view (**a**), whether the needle tip is located optimally should be confirmed by the A-P view (**b**). Note that the needle tip should be seen at the medial wall (point C) of the pedicle of the caudal vertebra, referring the axial view of MRI (**c**). Because the point C is just below the herniated mass, if we use this trajectory of the endoscopy, it brings us the easiest access to the mass

currently. When the cannula is set, the surgeon should pay attention not to injure the exiting nerve root. The cannula should be inserted with the bevel toward the exiting nerve root. In other words, when the oblique-type cannula is inserted, the longest side should be along with the endplate under the target disc. After the cannula is inserted into the disc, it should be rotated slowly, and the bevel would be toward the herniated mass (Fig. 3.3). Finally, the endoscope can be set.

3.2.4 How to Perform Discectomy

Discectomy is performed under desirable vision with perfusion of physiological saline. To ensure visibility, coagulate the damaged annulus nucleus/fibrous

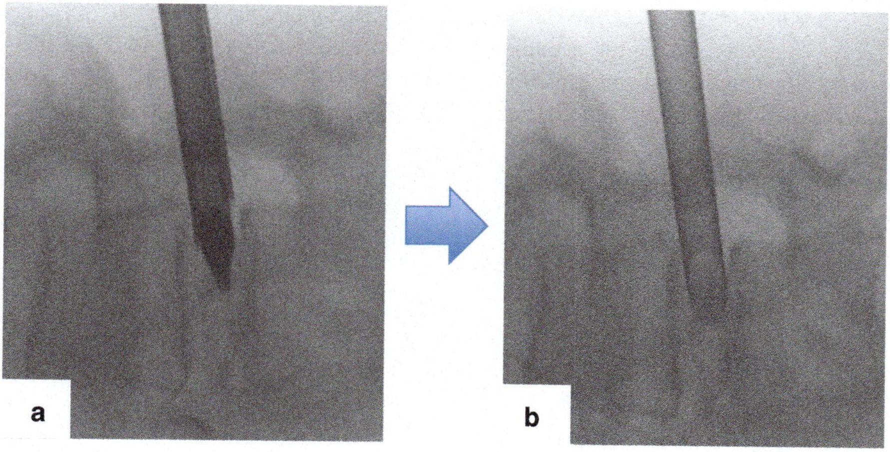

Fig. 3.3 An oblique-type cannula is set over the pencil-type obturator. Note that the cannula is inserted with the bevel toward the exiting nerve root. In other words, the longest side is inserted along with the endplate under the target disc to avoid injury to the exiting nerve (**a**). After the cannula is inserted into the disc safely, it is rotated slowly, and the bevel is toward the herniated mass (**b**)

Fig. 3.4 The upper half of the monitor screen presenting the dura mater/traversing nerve root looks red, while the lower half presenting the disc has a white appearance across the posterior longitudinal ligament. This view is called as "Half and half view"

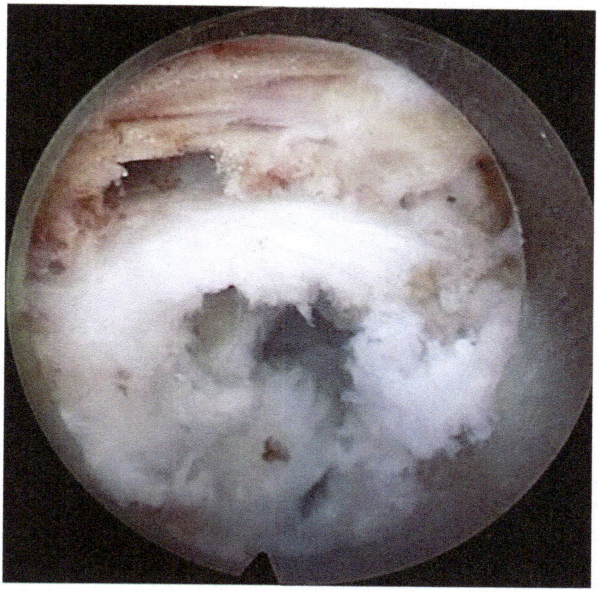

pulposus appropriately using radiofrequency, and it should be done repeatedly. After removal of a certain mass, the inserted cannula is gradually drawn and brought closer until the epidural space can be identified, which is called as "Half and Half view" (Fig. 3.4).

After removal of a certain mass and the inserted cannula is drawn and brought closer, a space to move the cannula easily is secured. Using the "hand-down technique," the cannula is re-inserted more horizontally under the herniated mass. Now, the base of the herniated mass is accessible. The mass is pulled out gradually.

Conflicts of Interest and Source of Funding None declared.

Sources of support: None.

Complications

4

Toru Maeda and Koichi Sairyo

Abstract

In this chapter, we describe surgery-related complications for transforaminal full-endoscopic surgery. Unlike the inter laminar approach, there are special complications such as exiting nerve root injury, seizure, etc. Surgeons should be aware of these complications and should pay attention to prevent the complications.

Keywords

Transforaminal approach · Full-endoscopic surgery · Local anesthesia · Complication · Exiting nerve injury

In the literature, many transforaminal (TF) full-endoscopic surgery-related complications have been reported. The TF approach utilizes Kambin's triangle [1–3] to access the spinal canal; thus, the surgical concept is absolutely different from the traditional interlaminar approach. For this reason, the surgical complication is assumed to be different from the one during interlaminar surgery. There are exiting nerve root injury, hematoma, intracranial hypertension, and so on.

4.1 Exiting Nerve Root Injury (ENRI)

Exiting nerve root injury, which is postoperative dysesthesia, is a typical complication during transforaminal surgery. As shown in Fig. 4.1, transforaminal surgery uses the Kambin's triangle to access into the canal. The superior aspect of the

---

T. Maeda · K. Sairyo (✉)
Department of Orthopedics, Tokushima University, Tokushima, Japan

K. Sairyo (ed.), *Transforaminal Full-Endoscopic Lumbar Surgery Under the Local Anesthesia*, https://doi.org/10.1007/978-981-15-7023-0_4

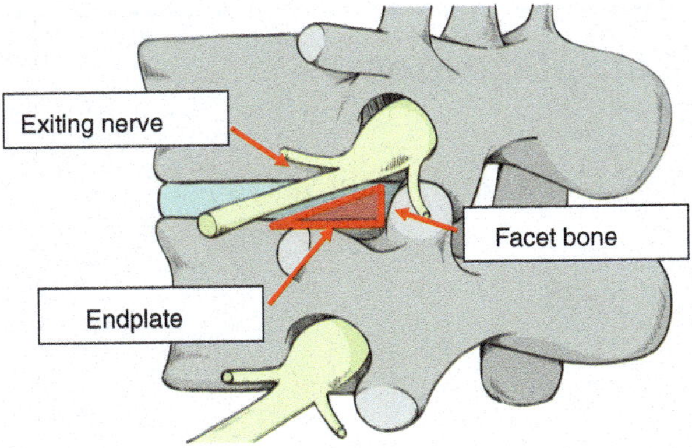

Fig. 4.1 Kambin triangle

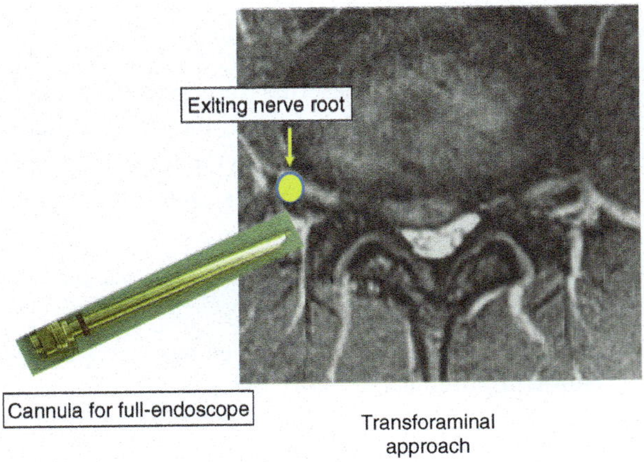

Fig. 4.2 Location of the exiting nerve and cannula

triangle is the exiting nerve root. Usually, traversing nerve root is covered by the facet joint. Thus, the nerve root injury is common in the exiting nerve compared to the traversing nerve. Figure 4.2 demonstrates the anatomical relationship between the cannula and the exiting nerve. The nerve is very close to the cannula. It has been reported that ENRI has occurred in 1.0–8.9% as reported in the literature [4]. In our early experience of 100 cases, we have 2% incidence of ENRI [5].

There are two possibilities to injure the exiting nerve root. The first possibility is direct injury by a cannula. When lidocaine infiltrates the exiting nerve root during local anesthesia, the patient does not feel any pain even though the nerve is injured. Under general or epidural anesthesia, the risk may increase. As a result dysesthesia and motor paresis would occur just after the surgery. With careful local anesthesia, this kind of complication can be avoided, and in our early 100 cases, no patient had such complication under local anesthesia [5].

The second type of ENRI is irritation of the dorsal root ganglion due to compression by the cannula wall during surgery. For such cases, leg dysesthesia would occur a couple of days after the surgery due to the swelling of the exiting nerve. There are

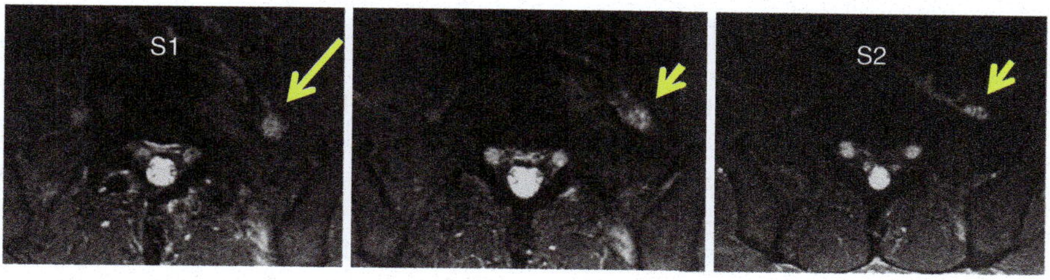

Fig. 4.3 Swelling of the exiting nerve after full-endoscopic surgery on STIR-MRI

two such cases among early 100 cases [5]. Both of them started complaining leg pain 2 days after the surgery. Figure 4.3 demonstrates MRI of the ENRI case. Immediately after the surgery, the leg pain disappeared. Two days after the surgery, he noticed leg paresthesia. The MRI indicates left L5 nerve root swelling and edema. With conservative treatment, the symptom disappeared.

4.2 Exiting Nerve Root Injury (ENRI) in the Fullendo KILF

In this section, we describe the ENRI during the full-endoscopic trans-Kambin triangle lumbar interbody fusion (fullendo KLIF). In this decade, the full-endoscopic technique has been applied to the interbody fusion through the Kambin triangle. Several authors reported their technique and named their own name. There are many names in the literature, although techniques are very similar to our fullendo-KLIF procedure. PELIF (percutaneous endoscopic LIF) [6], PETLIF (percutaneous endoscopic transforaminal LIF) [7], FELIF (full-endoscopic LIF) [8], and FETLIF (full-endoscopic transforaminal LIF) [9] have been used to describe the same method. Very recently, Lewandrowski et al. proposed lordotic endoscopic wedge lumbar interbody fusion (LEW-LIF) as the name for a similar technique [10]. We proposed full-endoscopic KLIF with the anatomical reason, since they all insert cages through the Kambin triangle [11].

The most common complication in the fullendo-KLIF would be ENRI. One can easily assume that a cage may damage the exiting nerve root, if Kambin triangle is small due to hypertrophy of the facet joint. The highest rate was reported by Lewandrowski et al. [10], and it was 60.4% (29/48), although most cases healed within 6 weeks of surgery. The second highest rate reported was 22% [12]. Abbasi et al. reported their technique called OLLIF, which is similar to KLIF. Their ENRI rate was as low as 5.3%, and they emphasized the important of intraoperative electrophysiological monitoring for the prevention of this complication [13]. Nagahama et al. [7] reported the rate to be 4.0%, and they also stated the importance of neural monitoring during the surgery. Actually, in our series, the first patient complained of ENRI, which was paresthesia in the anterior thigh (L4 dermatome) after fullendo-KLIF at L4/5. Presently, we have performed 16 cases; therefore, our ENRI rate was 6.25%. We also use electrophysiological monitoring during the surgery.

4.3 Post-Operative Hematoma

There are two types of post-operative hematoma: epidural and retroperitoneal hematoma [14]. Ahn et al. [14] performed transforaminal PED for 412 cases and experienced 4 (0.97%) cases with symptomatic retroperitoneal hematoma. In two cases, the volume was over 500 (ml), i.e., 1274 and 704 (ml), and open evacuation was required by the general surgeon. Injury to the terminal branch of the lumbar artery would be the reason. In our series, we did not experience such hematoma, but postsurgical epidural hematoma in 1 case (1%), which is common in the traditional spine surgery [5]. According to the National Survey on Japan in 2018, there was only one epidural hematoma among 1296 cases, less than 0.1%, meaning very rare complication [15].

4.4 Intracranial Hypertension (Seizure)

This is a very unique complication, and it must never occur during traditional open surgery, because it may be related to the water irrigation system during the full-endoscopic surgery. Intracranial hypertension during surgery may cause neck pain, headache, and seizure. Choi et al. [16] reported four cases of seizure among 16.725 cases of full-endoscopic surgery. Regarding the initial three cases, the seizure began 130, 80, and 110 min after the procedure had started. Thus, prolonged operation time may be a risk factor for those with seizure. Zhou et al. [17] had a case of intra-operative seizure among 426 full-endoscopic surgery. Mostly, they complained of neck pain before seizure; thus, it must be the indicator of the consequent seizure. Actually, Joh et al. [18] investigated the reason of the seizure by monitoring the cervical epidural pressure (EP) during full-endoscopic discectomy for 28 patients. Eight cases complained of neck pain, and high EP was monitored as the neck pain occurred. Cervical EP and intracranial pressure have a positive relationship; thus, when a patient complains of neck pain, intracranial pressure would be high. The intracranial hypertension may cause seizure. Indeed, in our earliest 100 cases, two patients complained of neck pain during surgery [5]. We completed surgery as soon as possible, and then we did not have any further complications such as seizure.

4.5 Dural Injury

Ishii reported the results of a nationwide survey of endoscopic surgery including 1296 transforaminal full-endoscopic surgery [15]. There are six cases with dural injury, and its incidence is 0.5% being very rare. In my initial 100 cases, there was no dural injury. So far, in my over 400 cases of the transforaminal approach, no dural injury has been experienced. Actually, our group has been mainly performing the inside-out technique [19–21]. As compared to the outside-in technique [22], there is no chance to touch the dural matter during the surgery. Thus, we have never experienced cases with dural injury during the transforaminal full-endoscopic surgery.

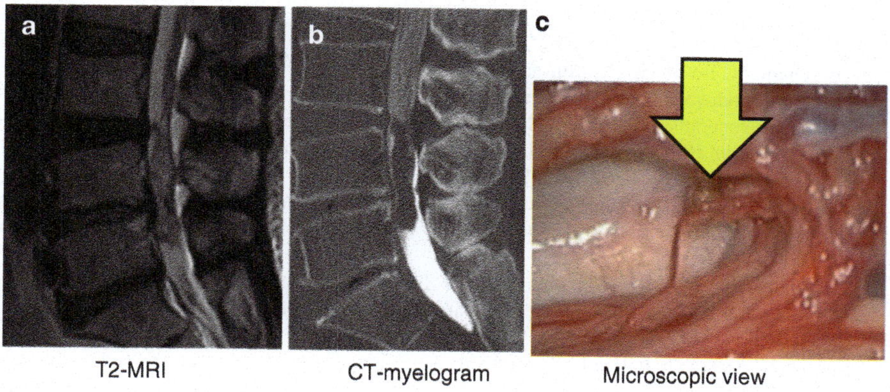

Fig. 4.4 Intradural herniated nucleus pulposus through the dural hole that had occurred during the previous full-endoscopic surgery. (**a**) T2 MRI. Large tumorous condition is seen at the level of L4 and L5 vertebral body. (**b**) Sagittal CT myelogram. Large tumorous mass is seen at the intradural space. (**c**) Microscopic view. Ther is a hole on the ventral aspect of the dura matter. An yellow arrow iondicates the hole of the dura matter

Our group has a very interesting case of dural injury [23]. The case was diagnosed as having intra-dural tumor before the surgery (Fig. 4.4a, b); thus, durotomy following laminectomy was performed. The mass was the herniated nucleus pulposus, and dural hole was found just at the ventral aspect of the mass (Fig. 4.4c; yellow allow). The patient had a history of transforaminal full-endoscopic discectomy at another hospital. We consulted the former hospital and got information of the dural tear during the surgery. After the surgery, disc material might herniate again and penetrate into the dural tube through the dural hole.

4.6 Conclusion

There are several complications in performing transforaminal full-endoscopic surgery. Surgeons should be aware of the complications and should focus on prevention.

References

1. Kambin P, Sampson S. Posterolateral percutaneous suction-excision of herniated lumbar intervertebral discs. Report of interim results. Clin Orthop Relat Res. 1986;207:37–43.
2. Kambin P, Brager MD. Percutaneous posterolateral discectomy. Anatomy and mechanism. Clin Orthop Relat Res. 1987;223:145–54.
3. Kambin P, Schaffer JL. Percutaneous lumbar discectomy. Review of 100 patients and current practice. Clin Orthop Relat Res. 1989;238:24–34.
4. Choi I, Ahn JO, So WS, Lee SJ, Choi IJ, Kim H. Exiting root injury in transforaminal endoscopic discectomy: preoperative image considerations for safety. Eur Spine J. 2013;22(11):2481–7.
5. Sairyo K, Matsuura T, Higashino K, Sakai T, Takata Y, Goda Y, Suzue N, Hamada D, Goto T, Nishisho T, Sato R, Tsutsui T, Tonogai I, Mineta K. Surgery related complications in percutaneous endoscopic lumbar discectomy under local anesthesia. J Med Investig. 2014;61(3–4):264–9. Review.

6. Nakamura S, Taguchi M. Full percutaneous lumbar interbody fusion: technical note. J Neurol Surg A Cent Eur Neurosurg. 2017;78(6):601–6.
7. Nagahama K, Ito M, Abe Y, Murota E, Hiratsuka S, Takahata M. Early clinical results of percutaneous endoscopic transforaminal lumbar interbody fusion: a new modified technique for treating degenerative lumbar spondylolisthesis. Spine Surg Relat Res. 2018;3(4):327–34.
8. Youn MS, Shin JK, Goh TS, Lee JS. Full endoscopic lumbar interbody fusion (FELIF): technical note. Eur Spine J. 2018;27(8):1949–55.
9. Kamson S, Lu D, Sampson PD, Zhang Y. Full-endoscopic lumbar fusion outcomes in patients with minimal deformities: a retrospective study of data collected between 2011 and 2015. Pain Physician. 2019;22(1):75–88.
10. Lewandrowski KU, Ransom NA, Ramírez León JF, Yeung A. The concept for a standalone lordotic endoscopic wedge lumbar interbody fusion: the LEW-LIF. Neurospine. 2019;16(1):82–95.
11. Sairyo K, Maeda T. Fullendo-KLIF for the anatomical nomenclature of the full-endoscope guided lumbar interbody fusion through the Kambin triangle: PELIF, PETLIF, FELIF, FE-TLIF or KLIF? EC Orthopaedics. 2019;10(9):743–5.
12. Morgenstern C, Yue JJ, Morgenstern R. Full percutaneous transforaminal lumbar interbody fusion using the facet-sparing, Trans-Kambin approach. Clin Spine Surg. 2019;33:40. https://doi.org/10.1097/BSD.0000000000000827. [Epub ahead of print].
13. Abbasi A, Khaghany K, Orandi V, Abbasi H. Clinical and radiological outcomes of oblique lateral lumbar interbody fusion. Cureus. 2019;11(2):e4029.
14. Ahn Y, Kim JU, Lee BH, Lee SH, Park JD, Hong DH, Lee JH. Postoperative retroperitoneal hematoma following transforaminal percutaneous endoscopic lumbar discectomy. J Neurosurg Spine. 2009;10(6):595–602.
15. Ishii K. Current status of endoscopic spine surgery in Japan: January to December 2018. J Jpn Orthop Assoc. 2020;94:68–75. (in Japanese).
16. Choi G, Kang HY, Modi HN, Prada N, Nicolau RJ, Joh JY, Pan WJ, Lee SH. Risk of developing seizure after percutaneous endoscopic lumbar discectomy. J Spinal Disord Tech. 2011;24(2):83–92.
17. Zhou C, Zhang G, Panchal RR, Ren X, Xiang H, Xuexiao M, Chen X, Tongtong G, Hong W, Dixson AD. Unique complications of percutaneous endoscopic lumbar discectomy and percutaneous endoscopic interlaminar discectomy. Pain Physician. 2018;21(2):E105–12.
18. Joh JY, Choi G, Kong BJ, Park HS, Lee SH, Chang SH. Comparative study of neck pain in relation to increase of cervical epidural pressure during percutaneous endoscopic lumbar discectomy. Spine (Phila Pa 1976). 2009;34(19):2033–8.
19. Yeung AT. The evolution of percutaneous spinal endoscopy and discectomy: state of the art. Mt Sinai J Med. 2000;67:327–32.
20. Yeung AT, Tsou PM. Posterolateral endoscopic excision for lumbar disc herniation: surgical technique, outcome, and complications in 307 consecutive cases. Spine. 2002;27:722–31.
21. Yeung AT, Yeung CA. Minimally invasive techniques for the management of lumbar disc herniation. Orthop Clin North Am. 2007;38(3):363–72.
22. Yoshinari H, Tezuka F, Yamashita K, Manabe H, Hayashi F, Ishihama Y, Sugiura K, Takata Y, Sakai T, Maeda T, Sairyo K. Transforaminal full-endoscopic lumbar discectomy under local anesthesia in awake and aware conditions: the inside-out and outside-in techniques. Curr Rev Musculoskelet Med. 2019;12:311–7.
23. Tamaki Y, Sakai T, Miyagi R, Nakagawa T, Shimakawa T, Sairyo K, Chikawa T. Intradural lumbar disc herniation after percutaneous endoscopic lumbar discectomy: case report. J Neurosurg Spine. 2015;23(3):336–9.

Part II

Discectomy

Inside-Out Technique of Transforaminal Full-Endoscopic Lumbar Discectomy (TELD)

5

Fumitake Tezuka

Abstract

The inside-out technique of transforaminal full-endoscopic lumbar discectomy is a traditional technique, which was developed from percutaneous nucleotomy by Hijikata. Transforaminal approach can be done under local anesthesia, and there are great benefits. During the surgery, patients would be in awake and aware condition; thus, severe nerve root injury can be avoided. The surgical technique is easy to adopt by beginners compared to outside-in technique. However, it has some issues which we should pay attention to during surgery. If there would be exiting nerve root irritation when approaching to the disc, it is important not to hesitate to change for outside-in technique.

Keywords

TELD · Local anesthesia · Discogram · Inside-out · Half and half view

5.1 Introduction

The inside-out technique is the procedure to put the cannula into the disc and to remove a herniated nucleus pulposus from the disc [1]. This is the most traditional procedure in transforaminal approach through Kambin's safety triangle [2].

F. Tezuka (✉)
Department of Orthopedics, Tokushima University, Tokushima, Japan

K. Sairyo (ed.), *Transforaminal Full-Endoscopic Lumbar Surgery Under the Local Anesthesia*, https://doi.org/10.1007/978-981-15-7023-0_5

5.2 Surgical Indication and Contraindication for TELD

5.2.1 Indication

Lumbar intervertebral disc herniation (intracanal, foraminal, and extraforaminal type) at the L1–L2 to L4–L5 level, and L5–S1 level with low iliac crest.

5.2.2 Contraindication

1. Sequestration type
2. Extrusion type with highly down-/up-migrated herniation
3. L5–S1 level with high iliac crest

5.3 Surgical Procedure of TELD

5.3.1 Anesthesia

We highly recommend performing TELD under local anesthesia. Exiting nerve root injury during surgery is one of the serious complications when approaching Kambin's safety triangle; however, we can prevent the complication because patients can complain of the symptom derived from exiting nerve root irritation under awake and aware condition.

5.3.2 Position

TELD is conducted with the patient in the prone position on the standard spine frame available for intraoperative c-arm image intensifier. Chest-knee position can decrease lumbar lordosis.

5.3.3 Premedication

Hydroxyzine hydrochloride (25–50 mg) and pentazocine hydrochloride (7.5–15 mg) were administered intravenously for premedication followed by local anesthesia. We have to pay attention to vasovagal reflex in young patients when inserting the cannula into the disc. Then, we routinely monitor their heart rate and blood pressure and perform intravenous injection of atropine when the heart rate is under 60 beats per minute before starting TELD.

5.3.4 Discogram

Insertion point is planned by preoperative MRI axial image (Fig. 5.1a, b). Distance from the midline of patient's back (between spinous process and insertion point) is calculated. The puncture needle is inserted from the starting point checking the lateral view of c-arm image intensifier. About 10 mL of 1% lidocaine is injected to the subcutaneous tissue, thereafter 2 mL at the surface of facet joint and 2 mL just below the surface of the annulus fibrosus. When putting the puncture needle on the surface of the disc on the lateral view of c-arm image intensifier (Fig. 5.2a), appropriate position of the tip of the needle is located between the medial pedicle line on anterior-posterior (AP) view (Fig. 5.2b). When the needle is inserted into the center

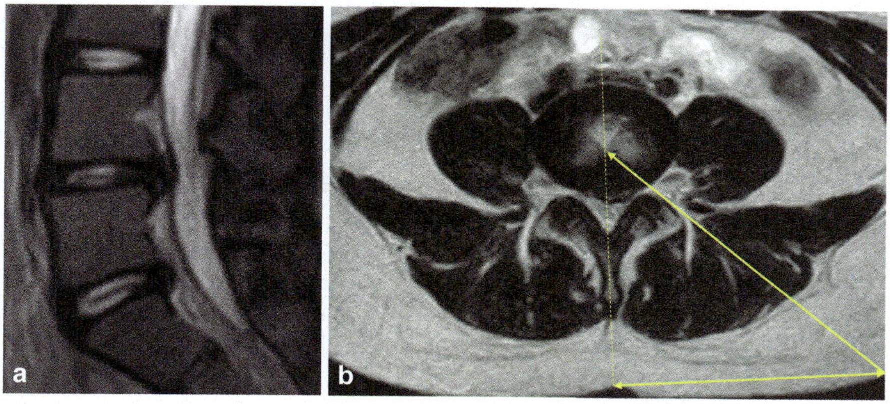

Fig. 5.1 L4/5 disc herniation in sagittal view of MRI T2WI (**a**), and axial view of MRI T2WI in the same case as (**a**); preoperative planning of the insertion point of puncture needle (**b**)

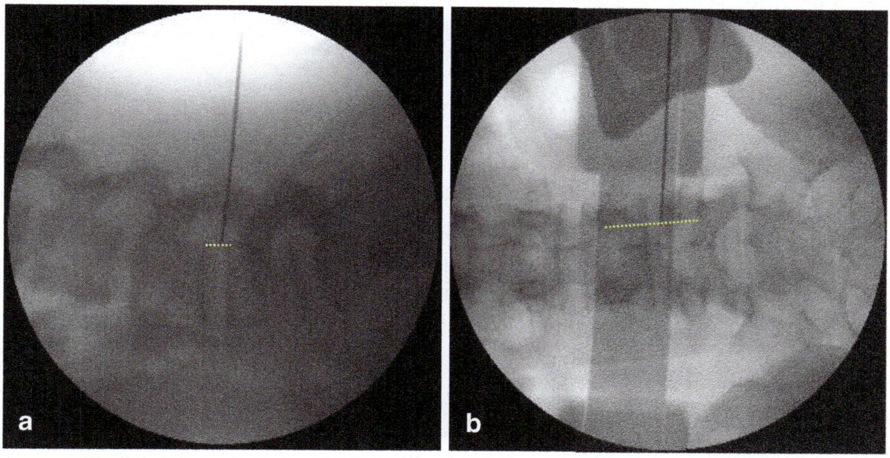

Fig. 5.2 Recommended puncture point of annulus fibrosus in lateral view (**a**), and in AP view (**b**)

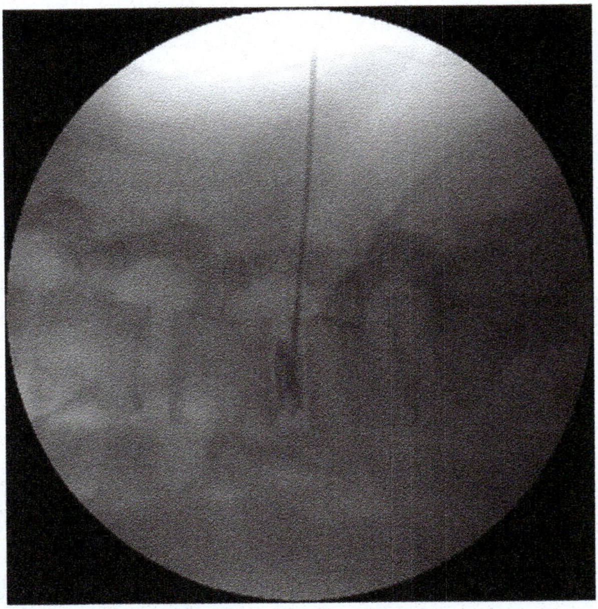

Fig. 5.3 Discogram shows posterior leakage of the contrast media

of the disc, we inject a mixture of contrast media and dye (indigo carmine) and make sure the posterior leakage of them checking the lateral view (Fig. 5.3). Indigo color can help to distinguish a herniated nucleus pulposus from annulus fibrosus and nerve roots.

5.3.5 Skin Incision, Insertion of the Endoscope

Skin incision of 8 mm is conducted and a guide pin is inserted into the disc through the puncture needle. Then, the obturator and cannula are inserted sequentially through the incision.

5.3.6 Discectomy

After inserting the cannula (Fig. 5.4a, b), we can start endoscopic viewing and remove the disc fragment at the base of the herniated mass, which are dyed indigo (Fig. 5.5b). The cannula is gradually moved toward the epidural space using the hand-down technique. When the herniated mass is removed, we can confirm pulsation of the dural sac and the traversing nerve root from the "half and half view," which consists of the borderline between the epidural space and disc space (Fig. 5.5b).

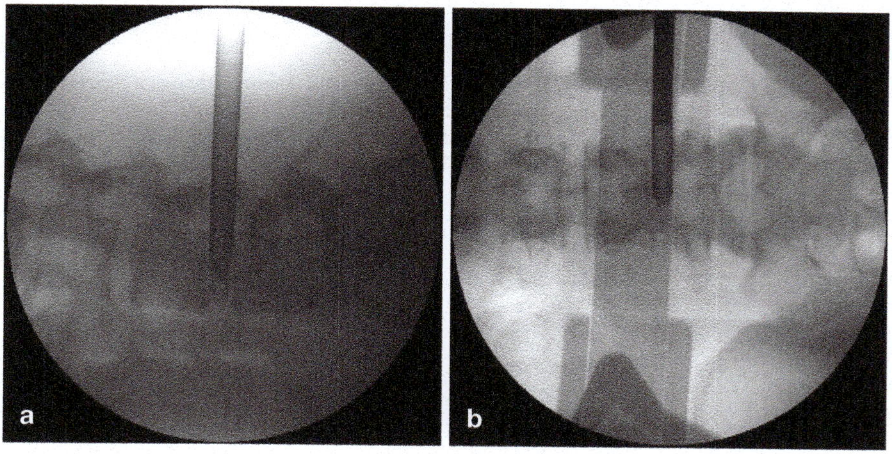

Fig. 5.4 Cannula is located in the intervertebral disc space (**a**, **b**)

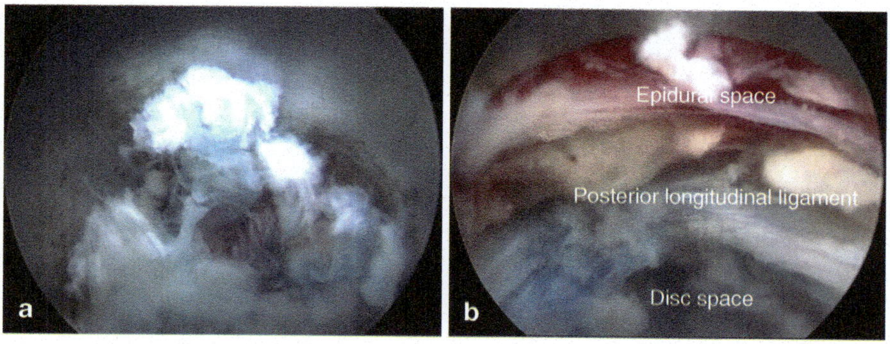

Fig. 5.5 Nucleus pulposus and herniated mass dyed indigo from the endoscopic viewing (**a**), and "half and half view" which consists of the borderline between the epidural space and disc space (**b**)

5.3.7 Wound Drainage and Skin Closure

We recommend leaving the drainage tube into the disc space to prevent postoperative hematoma. The subcutaneous tissue is closed by using an absorbable thread, and the skin is closed with a skin tape. The drainage tube can be removed the next morning.

Conflict of Interest and Source of Funding Nothing to be disclosed.

Sources of support: Nothing to be disclosed.

References

1. Sairyo K, Egawa H, Matsuura T, et al. State of the art: transforaminal approach for percutaneous endoscopic lumbar discectomy under local anesthesia. J Med Invest. 2014;61(3–4):217–25.
2. Kambin P, Schaffer JL. Percutaneous lumbar discectomy. Review of 100 patients and current practice. Clin Orthop Relat Res. 1989;238:23–34.

Outside-in Direct Fragmentectomy of TELD After Foraminoplasty

6

Tomoya Terai

Abstract

As a minimally invasive surgery for lumbar disc herniation, full-endoscopic discectomy (FED) is gaining attention. There are three types of FED, transforaminal and posterolateral method with local anesthesia and interlaminar method with epidural anesthesia and general anesthesia. There are two methods of transforaminal endoscopic lumbar discectomy (TELD) for accessing the lumbar intervertebral discs in transforaminal approach: "inside-out technique" and "outside-in technique." Following foraminoplasty, the cannula was moved into the epidural space with the outside-in technique. With epidural observation just beneath the nerve root, the extruded transligamentous fragment was confirmed. The direct fragmentectomy of TELD is possible from outside of the intradiscal space. In conclusion, the outside-in technique during the transforaminal approach for TELD is a useful and reliable technique to remove extruded transligamentous disc fragments. We describe the outside-in technique of TELD in this review.

Keywords

Lumbar disc herniation · Full-endoscopic discectomy · Local anesthesia Transforaminal approach · Outside-in technique

6.1 Introduction

Full-endoscopic discectomy (FED) for herniated nucleus pulposus (HNP) is a minimally invasive spine surgery and has recently become popular because of its minimal invasiveness, short-term hospitalization, and early rehabilitation [1–5]. There are three approaches to FED, the transforaminal approach (TF), the posterolateral

T. Terai (✉)
Department of Orthopedic Surgery, Shikoku Central Hospital, Shikokuchuo, Ehime, Japan

K. Sairyo (ed.), *Transforaminal Full-Endoscopic Lumbar Surgery Under the Local Anesthesia*, https://doi.org/10.1007/978-981-15-7023-0_6

approach (PL), and the interlaminar approach (IL) [5–8]. FED surgery is performed under general anesthesia, epidural anesthesia, and local anesthesia. The transforaminal endoscopic lumbar discectomy (TELD) in which we perform a resection of the intervertebral disc in the spinal canal under local anesthesia. The transforaminal method is a useful technique for cases in which general anesthesia is difficult or in cases where short-term hospitalization and early rehabilitation are desired.

There are two methods of TELD for accessing the lumbar intervertebral discs in transforaminal approach: "inside-out technique" and "outside-in technique" [9–11]. The most critical difference is the initial location of the endoscopic working cannula either inside the intervertebral disc or the foramen. In the inside-out method, the endoscope is first started by inserting into the intradiscal space after annulus fenestration. The nucleus pulposus is resected by observing the area directly below the HNPs from the intervertebral disc, and the endoscope is gradually pulled out of the intervertebral disc and moved toward the dorsal epidural space. It removes the HNPs just below the posterior longitudinal ligament or outside the disc. In the outside-in method, an endoscope is first started by placing the foramen outside the disc. The extruded disc fragments may be visualized in the epidural space through the transforaminal approach [12, 13]. It removes directly the fragments of HNP.

Exiting nerve root injury is likely to occur in cases with foraminal stenosis. Therefore, safely insert the cannula with the endoscope into the epidural space through the intervertebral foramen in patients with a foraminal stenosis. The foraminoplasty can be used to enlarge the intervertebral foramen, thereby avoiding exiting nerve root injury [14]. We describe the outside-in technique and direct fragmentectomy of TELD after foraminoplasty.

6.2 Surgical Procedure

6.2.1 Positioning and Skin Marking

All patients were placed in prone position on a radiolucent table. It planed the safest lateral starting point with a preoperative prone CT scan. Skin marking was done outward from spinous process.

6.2.2 Skin Incision and Local Anesthesia

The skin, subcutaneous tissues and lateral facet joint were infiltrated with 1% lignocaine for local anesthesia. A long needle was introduced under fluoroscopy, and the superior articular process (SAP) of the facet joint and pedicle checked its position in the lateral fluoroscopic view. The needle was manipulated further to reach the mid-pedicular line in AP view and posterior vertebral line in lateral view. 2 ml was injected into the annulus fibrosus. The total amount of local anesthesia was usually about 10–15 ml.

6.2.3 Needle Insertion and Discography

In this approach, a disc puncture was made along the outside of the SAP of the facet joint. The discography was performed with 2 ml of the solution (indigo carmine 2 ml + contrast agent 2 ml + 1% lignocaine 1 ml) after putting the needle further inside the disc.

6.2.4 Cannula Placement

In the outside-in technique, the cannula is placed on the disc surface and just outside of the intervertebral foramen. A guidewire was inserted, and the needle was removed and a serial dilator is used to gradually enlarge the annulus fibrosus. There are four dilators, and the number of dilators to be inserted into the disc is adjusted according to the disc height. Dilators that are difficult to insert are placed on the disc surface. The cannula is placed so that the tip of the cannula is inserted into the annulus of the intervertebral disc (Fig. 6.1). When the endoscope is inserted at the foramen, the outside of the facet joint can be observed (Fig. 6.2). It is easy to understand the

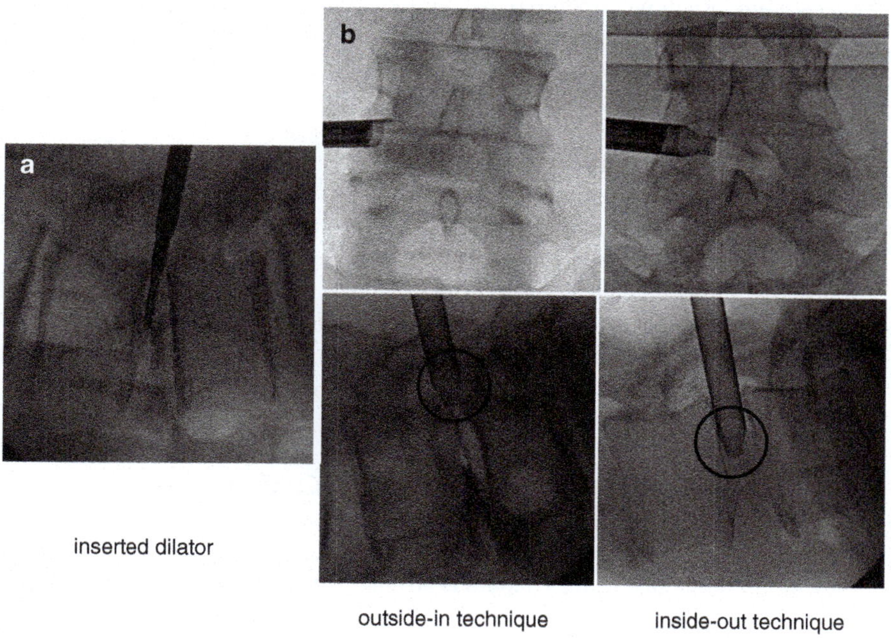

Fig. 6.1 (**a**) Two dilators inserted into the disc; the other two dilators are placed on the surface of the disc. (**b**) Starting position of the cannula during the outside-in and inside-out method. The location can be confirmed under C-arm fluoroscopic guidance

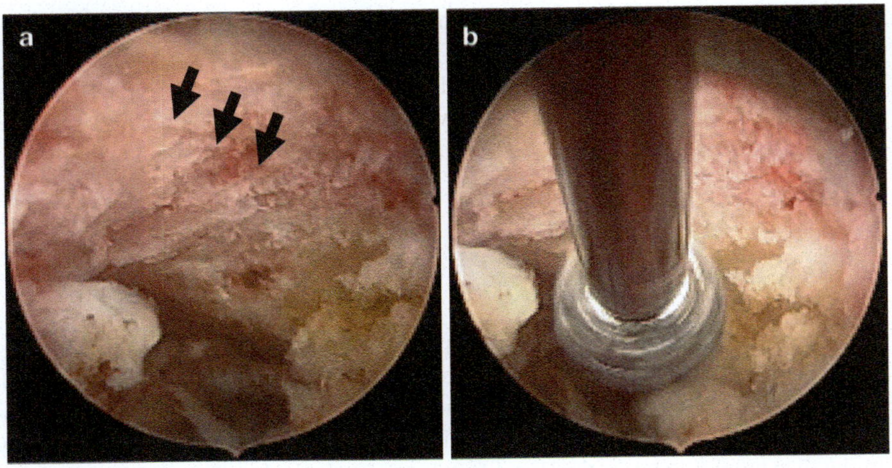

Fig. 6.2 Endoscopic views during surgery. (**a**) The endoscope was placed on the outside facet to visualize the lesion of SAP (black arrow). (**b**) Cutting SAP from outside with a high-speed drill

orientation, if we can observe the bony tissue of the foramen. We move away from the facet joint; it will be difficult to operate because it will be covered with soft tissue at the start of the endoscope, bleeding will increase, and the exiting nerve root will be closed.

6.2.5 Foraminoplasty

This technique would be enlargement of the neuroforamen for safer insertion of the cannula into the spinal canal using a high-speed drill, which is the best technique for this purpose. Following enlargement of the foramen, the cannula could be inserted without compressing the exiting nerve root. Figure 6.3 shows representative computed tomography (CT) scans before and after foraminoplasty. In the foraminal stenosis case, partial removal of the inferior facet and/or pediculotomy is often useful.

6.2.6 Ligamentum Flavum Resection and Confirmation of Traversing Nerve Root

Following foraminoplasty, the cannula is advanced into the intervertebral space. A disc stained blue can be observed, and it can be distinguished from the ligamentum flavum and the epidural space. To observe the traversing nerve root, the ligament flavum attached to the lateral recess is peeled off from the bone and resect to confirm the epidural fat and traversing nerve root in the spinal canal (Fig. 6.4).

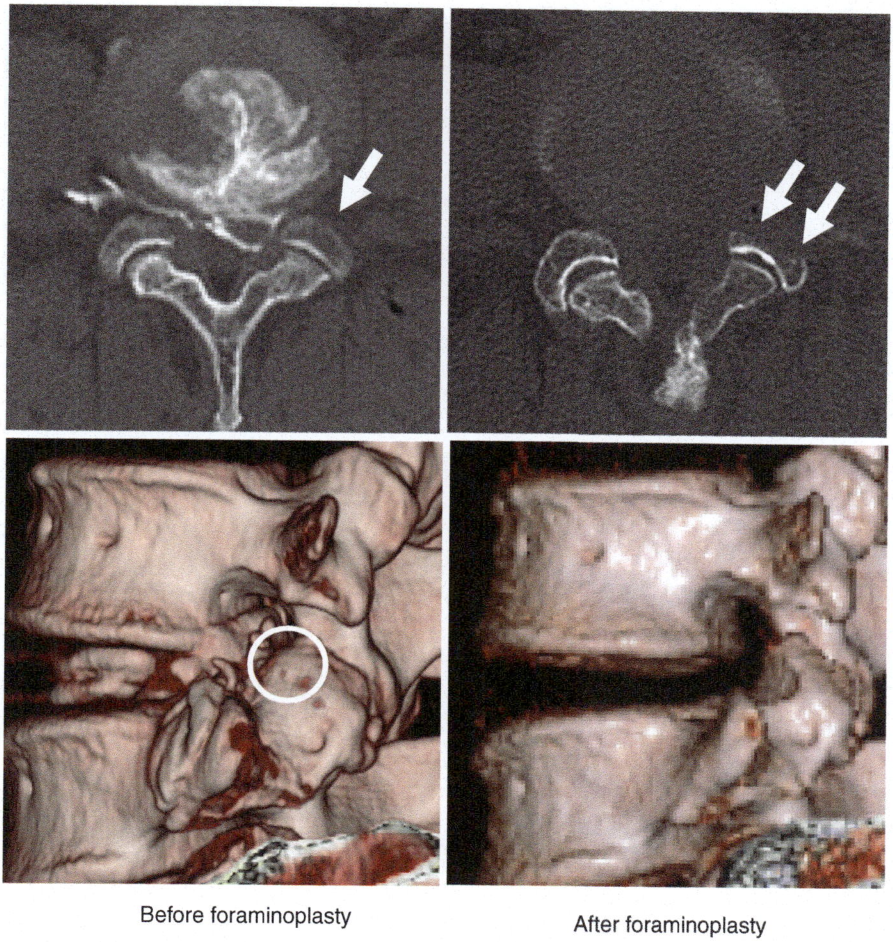

Fig. 6.3 CT scan shows that intervertebral foramen before and after foraminoplasty. After cutting the tip of the SAP, the narrow foramen became enlarged

6.2.7 Ventral Epiduroscopy and Herniotomy

The epiduroscopic observation technique can observe the herniated fragments from the ventral epidural space. A cannula of duck-bill type is commonly used for the transforaminal FED procedure. During the inside-out technique, the long wall aspect is on the ventral side, whereas during the epiduroscopic observation it is dorsal. The longer wall of the cannula is placed against the neural tissue, including the traversing nerve root and dura mater. Thus, this technique is safe and reliable for the removal of migrated fragments in the epidural space. HNPs inside of the canal would become visible and direct fragmentectomy is then possible from the outside of the canal (Fig. 6.5).

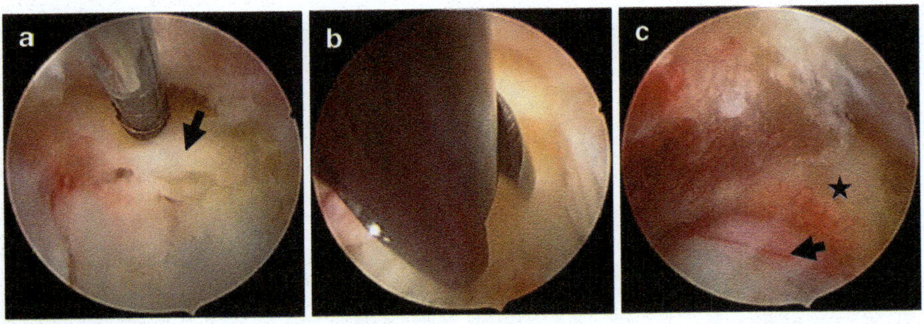

Fig. 6.4 (**a**) Boundary between SAP and ligamentum flavum (black arrow). (**b**) The ligamentum flavum removed with a punch. (**c**) Excision of ligament flavum allows observation of epidural fat tissue (black star) and traversing nerve root (black arrow)

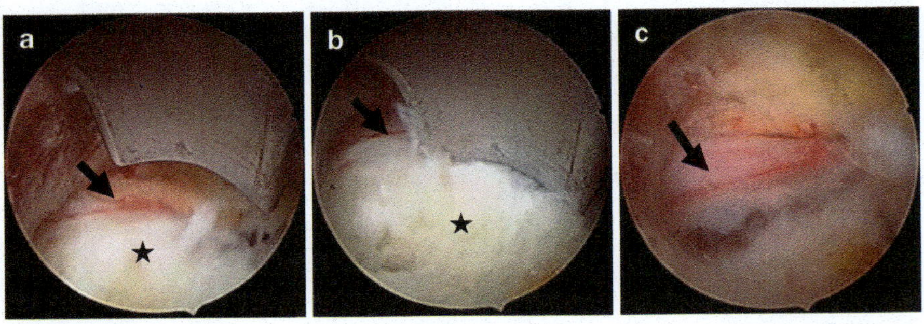

Fig. 6.5 (**a**) The herniation fragment can be observed on the ventral side of the traversing nerve root. (**b**) The longer side of the cannula is placed into the dorsal aspect to protect the nerve root and remove the HNP fragment. (**c**) Decompression of traversing nerve root can be confirmed: traversing nerve root (black arrow), herniation (black star)

6.2.8 Hemostasis

Hemostasis was achieved by the curved radiofrequency probe, which was also used as a probe for the search for hidden fragments. If the blood pressure is high, reduce the blood pressure or increase the water pressure of the reflux liquid to stop the bleeding and secure the visual field.

6.3 Advantage and Disadvantage of Inside-Out and Outside-In Technique

In the inside-out method, endoscopic operation is started from the intradiscal space, so there is little bleeding and nerve damage is less likely to occur, and it is considered to be the safest procedure at the beginning of TELD. However, the patient may complain of severe back pain when inserting a pencil dilator or cannula into the disc space under local anesthesia.

In the outside-in method, it is possible to remove the nucleus pulposus without approaching the intradiscal space, and the pressure in the intervertebral disc is reduced. This can reduce low back pain when inserting the serial dilator and cannula into the intervertebral disc under local anesthesia during the approach. Resection of the nucleus pulposus and herniation can be added while looking inside the disc. However, some bone resection with foraminoplasty is required to insert the cannula and there is a learning curve.

6.4 Complication of TELD

The complication of TELD is exiting nerve root injury. Causes include direct injury during approach, compression by intraoperative manipulation of cannula, and post-operative hematoma. TELD under local anesthesia allows direct monitoring of nerve root irritation during surgery, thus avoiding direct damage. In addition, by the foraminoplasty and the outside-in method, it is possible to avoid exiting nerve root injury due to cannula compression. TELD approaches from the lateral side, so there is a risk of abdominal organ injury and retroperitoneal hematoma, and it is necessary to confirm the position of the organ in the preoperative plan. In the case of FED, the epidural pressure is increased due to the use of the perfusate, and seizures due to elevated cerebral pressure have been reported [15–17].

6.5 Discussion

The great efforts by Yeung et al. [1–3], established the current system of transforaminal FED. In Japan, Dezawa et al. [4, 7, 8, 18, 19] developed new devices for FED, such as an ultrathin high-speed drill and contributed to further development of the FED procedure. We utilized two additional techniques to remove the direct fragment in the epidural space: epiduroscopic observation and foraminoplasty [12].

A contained HNP is a good indication for removal by a simple transforaminal approach with the inside-out technique. However, with transligamentous, extruded, or sequestration types, complete removal is difficult. In such situations, we need additional techniques. The interlaminar approach [4] and translaminar technique [7] are good options, but these cannot be performed under local anesthesia. The transforaminal epiduroscopic observation technique is the other option. It can be conducted under local anesthesia and performed via a transforaminal approach. Using this technique, one can observe the herniated fragments from the ventral epidural space. This technique enables observation of the central portion of the spinal canal.

Too much retraction of neural tissue may cause palsy. In the literature, many FED-related complications have been reported. Exiting nerve root injury is a particular complication in the transforaminal approach. The most beneficial aspect of the transforaminal epiduroscopic observation procedure is that it can be conducted under local anesthesia. During the operation, the patient may feel pain and numbness and can complain if any develops. Thus, this technique is safe and reliable for direct fragmentectomy in the epidural space with local anesthesia. However, there is one limitation in the narrow foramen case. If the 8-mm cannula is inserted through the narrow foramen, the cannula may compress the exiting nerve root, leading to palsy. For such cases, foraminoplasty is necessary to safely insert the cannula into the epidural space.

The technique of foraminoplasty is SAP resection to enlarge the foramen using a high-speed drill. Following enlargement of the foramen, the cannula could be inserted without compressing the exiting nerve root. Lee et al. [20] showed that foraminoplasty is essential to avoid injuring the exiting nerve root by insertion of the cannula through the narrow foramen.

Some authors reported the literature on outside-in technique with transforaminal approach [10–12]. This technique enabled the surgeon to visualize the traversing nerve root and HNP. Lewandrowski reviewed that the outside-in method may be more appropriate for foraminal lateral recess stenosis that is primarily caused by facet joint hypertrophy and upward migration of the SAP [21].

6.6 Conclusion

In this chapter, we described TELD procedures using the outside-in technique of FED. The FED surgery only requires an 8 mm skin incision and is the minimally invasive disc surgery. For the outside-in method, SAP resection with foraminoplasty is an important technique. The outside-in method is considered to be a very useful technique in FED surgery under local anesthesia for reducing pain when approaching to the disc. FED under local anesthesia would be of benefit for elderly patients and would be more popular in the future. We should master both the outside-in and inside-out techniques of TELD.

References

1. Yeung AT. The evolution of percutaneous spinal endoscopy and discectomy: state of the art. Mt Sinai J Med. 2000;67:327–32.
2. Yeung AT, Tsou PM. Posterolateral endoscopic excision for lumbar disc herniation: surgical technique, outcome, and complications in 307 consecutive cases. Spine. 2002;27:722–31.
3. Yeung AT, Yeung CA. Minimally invasive techniques for the management of lumbar disc herniation. Orthop Clin North Am. 2007;38(3):363–72.
4. Dezawa A, Sairyo K. New minimally invasive endoscopic discectomy technique through the interlaminar space using a percutaneous endoscope. Asian J Endosc Surg. 2011;4(2):94–8.
5. Sairyo K, Egawa H, Matsuura T, Takahashi M, Higashino K, Sakai T, et al. State of the art: transforaminal approach for percutaneous endoscopic lumbar discectomy under local anesthesia. J Med Investig. 2014;61(3–4):217–25.
6. Ruetten S, Komp M, Merk H, Godolias G. Use of newly developed instruments and endoscopes: full-endoscopic resection of lumbar disc herniations via the interlaminar and lateral transforaminal approach. J Neurosurg Spine. 2007;6(6):521–30.

7. Dezawa A, Mikami H, Sairyo K. Percutaneous endoscopic translaminar approach for herniated nucleus pulposus in the hidden zone of the lumbar spine. Asian J Endosc Surg. 2011;5(4):200–3.
8. Koga S, Sairyo K, Shibuya I, Kanamori Y, Kosugi T, Matsumoto H, et al. Minimally invasive removal of a recurrent lumbar herniated nucleus pulposus by the small incised microendoscopic discectomy interlaminar approach. Asian J Endosc Surg. 2012;5(1):34–7.
9. Gore S, Yeung A. The "inside out" transforaminal technique to treat lumbar spinal pain in an awake and aware patient under local anesthesia: results and a review of the literature. Int J Spine Surg. 2014;8:28.
10. Kim HS, Adsul N, Kim KJ, Jang JS, Jang IT, Oh SH. Get ready for 100 years of active spine life using percutaneous endoscopic spine surgery (PESS). J Minim Invasive Spine Surg Tech. 2018;3(1):1–8.
11. Yoshinari H, Tezuka F, Yamashita K, Manabe H, Hayashi F, Ishihama Y, et al. Transforaminal full-endoscopic lumbar discectomy under local anesthesia in awake and aware condition: the inside-out and outside-in techniques. Curr Rev Musculoskelet Med. 2019;12(3):311–7.
12. Henmi T, Terai T, Hibino N, Yoshioka S, Kondo K, Goda Y, et al. Percutaneous endoscopic lumbar discectomy utilizing ventral epiduroscopic observation technique and foraminoplasty for transligamentous extruded nucleus pulposus: technical note. J Neurosurg Spine. 2016;24(2):275–80.
13. Sairyo K, Chikawa T, Nagamachi A. State-of-the-art transforaminal percutaneous endoscopic lumbar surgery under local anesthesia: discectomy, foraminoplasty, and ventral facetectomy. J Orthop Sci. 2018;23(2):229–36.
14. Henmi T, Terai T, Nagamachi A, Sairyo K. Morphometric changes of the lumbar intervertebral foramen after percutaneous endoscopic foraminoplasty under local anesthesia. J Neurol Surg A Cent Eur Neurosurg. 2018;79(1):19–24.
15. Choi G, Kang HY, Modi HN, Prada N, Nicolau RJ, Joh JY, et al. Risk of developing seizure after percutaneous endoscopic lumbar discectomy. J Spinal Disord Tech. 2011;24(2):83–92.
16. Choi I, Ahn JO, So WS, Lee SJ, Choi IJ, Kim H. Exiting root injury in transforaminal endoscopic discectomy: preoperative image considerations for safety. Eur Spine J. 2013;22(11):2481–7.
17. Sairyo K, Matsuura T, Higashino K, Sakai T, Takata Y, Goda Y, et al. Surgery related complications in percutaneous endoscopic lumbar discectomy under local anesthesia. J Med Investig. 2014;61(3–4):264–9.
18. Kitahama Y, Sairyo K, Dezawa A. Percutaneous endoscopic transforaminal approach to decompress the lateral recess in an elderly patient with spinal canal stenosis, herniated nucleus pulposus and pulmonary comorbidities. Asian J Endosc Surg. 2013;6(2):130–3.
19. Sairyo K, Kitagawa Y, Dezawa A. Percutaneous endoscopic discectomy and thermal annuloplasty for professional athletes. Asian J Endosc Surg. 2013;6(4):292–7.
20. Lee SH, Kang HS, Choi G, Kong BJ, Ahn Y, Kim JS, et al. Foraminoplastic ventral epidural approach for removal of extruded herniated fragment at the L5–S1 level. Neurol Med Chir (Tokyo). 2010;50(12):1074–8.
21. Lewandrowski KU. "Outside-in" technique, clinical results, and indications with transforaminal lumbar endoscopic surgery: a retrospective study on 220 patients on applied radiographic classification of foraminal spinal stenosis. Int J Spine Surg. 2014;8:26.

TELD for High School Athletes

7

Fumitake Tezuka

Abstract

In general, young athletes diagnosed as having lumbar disc herniation are treated conservatively. However, most patients have limited time, just 3 years as high school students. Because they may miss the chance of returning to their sports activity, we should show them the plan including operative or nonoperative treatment and the period required for returning to play their sports activity as soon as possible. Transforaminal full-endoscopic lumbar discectomy under local anesthesia can be one of the promising procedures for young athletes.

Keywords

High school athletes · Lumbar disc herniation · TELD · Return to play · Sports activity

7.1 Introduction

Lumbar disc herniation is prevalent comparatively in young individuals. Surgical intervention is sometimes required in young athletes for an early return to their sports activity. Transforaminal full-endoscopic lumbar discectomy (TELD) is the least invasive lumbar disc surgery, which can be performed under local anesthesia and requires only an 8 mm skin incision and minimal disruption of the back muscles. It is very beneficial merit for high school athletes as they can return to their sports activities and also study.

F. Tezuka (✉)
Department of Orthopedics, Tokushima University, Tokushima, Japan

K. Sairyo (ed.), *Transforaminal Full-Endoscopic Lumbar Surgery Under the Local Anesthesia*, https://doi.org/10.1007/978-981-15-7023-0_7

7.2 Surgical Indications and Contraindications for TELD

These are same as for adults. Patients need to be able to understand the pros and cons of this procedure and need to be in prone position during surgery under local anesthesia. Then, we routinely check the preoperative discogram prior to their surgery in outpatient clinic and demonstrate to insert a puncture needle into the intervertebral disc space as the first step of TELD.

7.3 Surgical Procedure of TELD

Steps of anesthesia, position, and premedication are described in Chaps. 5 and 6. Disc degeneration of high school students is not severe and intervertebral disc pressure is very high. We usually pay attention to vasovagal reflex due to pain in especially young patients like high school students when inserting the cannula into the disc by using the "inside-out" technique. Then, we routinely monitor their heart rate and blood pressure and perform intravenous injection of atropine prior to surgery when the heart rate is under 60 beats per minute. And, we highly recommend the "outside-in" technique to decrease intervertebral disc pressure.

7.4 Case Series

We experienced 16 patients (12 men and 4 women), who underwent TELD for lumbar disc herniation and lumbar discogenic pain with high signal intensity zone (HIZ) in T2 weighted image of lumbar MRI. Their average age was 16.6 years (15–18 years old). We retrospectively evaluated sports activity, duration between symptom onset and visit to our hospital, affected disc level, perioperative complications, and return to play their sports activity. They played baseball (5 patients), softball (2), basketball (2), track and field (2), rugby (1), American football (1), soccer (1), handball (1), and boxing (1). Average duration until visiting our hospital was 8.4 months (1–26 months). All patients underwent TELD under local anesthesia. Four patients who were diagnosed as having lumbar discogenic pain underwent additional thermal annuloplasty. The affected disc levels were L4–L5 for 12 patients, L5–S1 for 2 patients, and simultaneous 2 level TELD (L3–L4 and L4–L5, L4–L5 andd L5–S1) for 2 patients. There were no perioperative complications such as exiting nerve root injury. Two patients were excluded who had already retired due to pain until they visited our hospital, and 13 of 14 patients could return to play their sports activity (92.9%). The average period required for returning to play sports activity was 7 weeks (4–8 weeks). These results are not inferior to previous studies which were treated by microdiscectomy (Table 7.1).

Table 7.1 Surgical treatment and return to play patients' original sports activities

First author	Year	Case	Age	Operation	Return to play (%)	(week)
Watkins [1]	2012	75	28.1	Microdiscectomy	89	23.2
Earhart [2]	2013	40	32.2	Microdiscectomy	97.5	34.8
Yoshimoto [3]	2013	23	19.4	Microdiscectomy	82.6	10.8
Our case series	2018	16	16.6	TELD	92.9	7

7.5 Conclusion

In general, young athletes diagnosed as having lumbar disc disease are also treated conservatively by taking analgesics, epidural steroid injection, physical therapy, and activity modification. However, most patients have limited time, just 3 years as high school students. From the result of duration until they visited our hospital, it took long time for them. Because they may miss the chance of returning to their sports activity, we should show them the plan including operative or nonoperative treatment and the period required for returning to play their sports activity as soon as possible.

Conflict of Interest and Source of Funding Nothing to be disclosed.
Sources of support: Nothing to be disclosed.

References

1. Watkins RG IV, Hanna R, Chang D, Watkins RG III. Return-to-play outcomes after microscopic lumbar diskectomy in professional athletes. Am J Sports Med. 2012;40:2530–5.
2. Earhart JS, Roberts D, Roc G, Gryzlo S, Hsu W. Effects of lumbar disk herniation on the careers of professional baseball players. Orthopedics. 2012;35:43–9.
3. Yoshimoto M, Takebayashi T, Ida K, Tanimoto K, Yamashita T. Microendoscopic discectomy in athletes. J Orthop Sci. 2013;18:902–8.

Transforaminal Approach for L5-s Level

8

Fumitake Tezuka

Abstract

The trajectory of TELD can be limited by the surrounding anatomical structure. TELD for the central-type lumbar disc herniation at the L5-s disc level is more technically demanding than TELD at the L4–L5 disc level because of the interference of the iliac crest. However, in the clinical setting, such anatomical particularities can be overcome by using a hand-down technique with the possible addition of a foraminoplasty when we perform TELD at the L5-s disc level.

Keywords

Lumbar disc herniation · L5-s intervertebral disc · TELD · Iliac crest Foraminoplasty

8.1 Introduction

From the results of anatomical study using CT images, the trajectory of transforaminal full-endoscopic lumbar discectomy (TELD) at the L5-s disc level is limited by the surrounding anatomical structure such as the iliac crest [1]. In general, full-endoscopic discectomy using an interlaminar approach [2, 3], microendoscopic discectomy [4, 5], or conventional open discectomy under general anesthesia can resolve this problem in cases of L5-s disc herniation with a high iliac crest. However, in patients without high iliac crest, TELD can be one of the possible surgical options of lumbar disc herniation at the L5-s disc level.

F. Tezuka (✉)
Department of Orthopedics, Tokushima University, Tokushima, Japan

K. Sairyo (ed.), *Transforaminal Full-Endoscopic Lumbar Surgery Under the Local Anesthesia*, https://doi.org/10.1007/978-981-15-7023-0_8

8.2 Preoperative Planning of TELD at L5-s Disc Level

Extraforaminal type and foraminal type of disc herniation are easier to be treated by TELD. On the other hand, in the case of intracanal type L5-s disc herniation, operability of TELD depends on the location of both herniated nucleus pulposus (HNP) and iliac crest. Because the height of the iliac crest cannot be assessed by only lateral view of plain X-ray of the lumbar spine, we recommend to check preoperative discogram and CT discogram (CTD). CTD can help to understand the three-dimensional relationship between HNP and bony structures such as the iliac crest and superior articular process and to make the preoperative plan of the trajectory of TELD (Fig. 8.1).

8.3 Surgical Procedure of TELD

Steps of anesthesia, position, and premedication are described in other chapters. We highly recommend "outside-in" technique and foraminoplasty when performing TELD at the L5-s disc level. After putting the cannula into the intervertebral foramen, we can start foraminoplasty by using a high-speed drill which results in widening the Kambin's safety triangle and getting closer to HNP (Fig. 8.2).

Figure 8.3a shows the endoscopic view during foraminoplasty; a part of HNP dyed by indigo carmine can be found behind the superior articular process. After direct fragmentectomy of TELD with foraminoplasty, we can see "half and half" view and make sure decompressed S1 traversing nerve root (Fig. 8.3b).

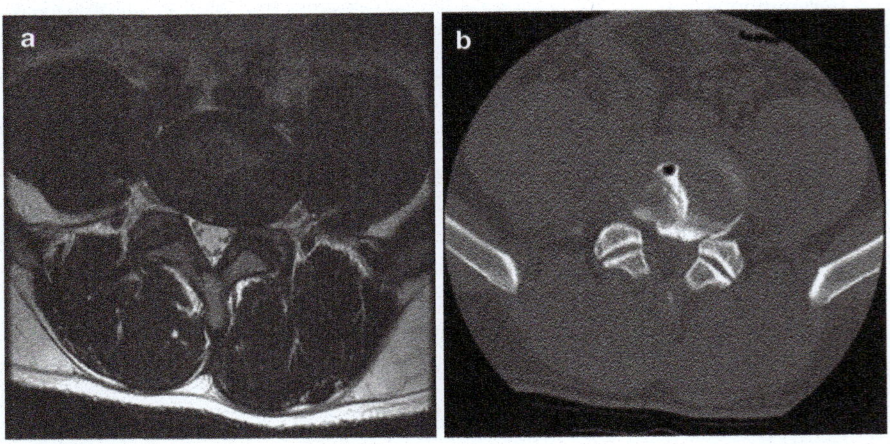

Fig. 8.1 (**a**) Preoperative axial image of MRI, T2WI. Intracanal type disc herniation at L5-s disc level, left side. (**b**) Preoperative reconstructed CTD shows anatomical relationship between HNP and surrounding bony structures

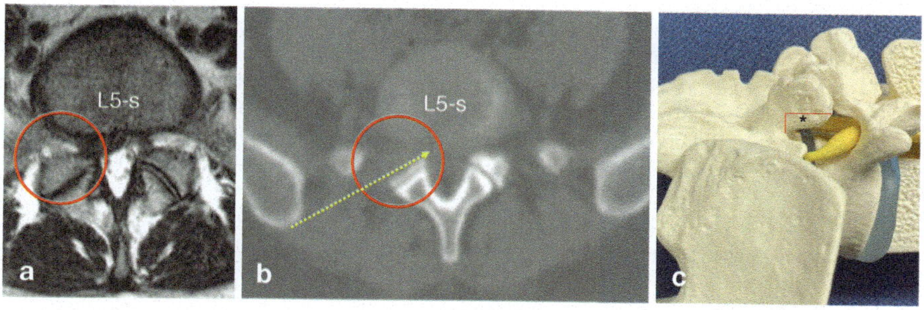

Fig. 8.2 (**a**) Preoperative axial image of MRI, T2WI. Intracanal type disc herniation at L5-s disc level, right side. Red circle indicates preoperative thickness of superior articular process (SAP). (**b**) Postoperative reconstructed CT image after TELD with foraminoplasty. Red circle indicates thinner thickness of SAP after foraminoplasty, and yellow arrow indicates trajectory line which could directly access HNP. (**c**) Asterisk (*) indicates schematic cutting area of foraminoplasty

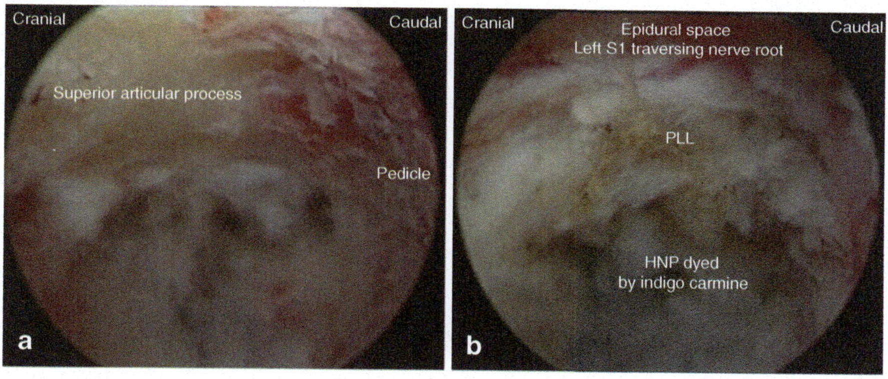

Fig. 8.3 (**a**) Endoscopic view during foraminoplasty. (**b**) Endoscopic half and half view after TELD with foraminoplasty

8.4 Conclusion

The maximum inclination angle indicates that TELD for the central type of LDH at the L5–S1 disc level is more technically demanding than TELD at the L4–L5 disc level because of the interference of the iliac crest. However, in the clinical setting, such anatomical particularities can be overcome by using a hand-down technique with the possible addition of a foraminoplasty when we perform TELD at the L5–S1 disc level.

Conflict of Interest and Source of Funding Nothing to be disclosed.

Sources of support: Nothing to be disclosed.

References

1. Tezuka F, Sakai T, Abe M, et al. Anatomical considerations of the iliac crest on percutaneous endoscopic discectomy using a transforaminal approach. Spine J. 2017;17(12):1875–80.
2. Choi G, Lee SH, Raiturker PP, et al. Percutaneous endoscopic interlaminar discectomy for intracanalicular disc herniations at L5–S1 using rigid working channel endoscope. Neurosurgery. 2006;58:ONS59–68.
3. Dezawa A, Sairyo K. New minimally invasive endoscopic discectomy technique through the interlaminar space using a percutaneous foraminoscope. Asian J Endosc Surg. 2011;4:94–8.
4. Foley KT, Smith MM. Microendoscopic discectomy. Tech Neurosurg. 1997;3:301–7.
5. Destandeau J. Technical features of endoscopic surgery for lumbar disc herniation: 191 patients. Neurochirurgie. 2004;50:6–10.

Part III

Decompression for Lumbar Spinal Canal Stenosis

9 Full-Endoscopic Foraminoplasty/ Foraminotomy for Foraminal Stenosis

Kazuta Yamashita

Abstract

Lumbar foraminal stenosis at the lumbosacral junction is particularly significant because it tends to cause severe pain and neurological dysfunction due to its anatomical features. The minimally invasive full-endoscopic lumbar foraminoplasty (FELF) without fusion is a modification of transforaminal full-endoscopic discectomy. It is possible to perform FELF under local anesthesia. FELF is performed through an 8 mm skin incision and damage to the paravertebral muscles is minimal; this technique is thus the least invasive lumbar surgery for lumbar foraminal stenosis available at this time.

The lumbar intervertebral foramen is a space that contains the spinal nerve and dorsal root ganglia. The pathology of lumbar foraminal stenosis was first reported in 1927 [1, 2] as one of possible origins of sciatica. The concept of lumbar foraminal stenosis had been defined as one of the lateral spinal stenoses [3]. Clinical lumbar foraminal stenosis is often unrecognized and accounts for approximately 60% of failed back surgery syndromes with continued postoperative symptoms [4]. Lumbar foraminal stenosis at the lumbosacral junction is particularly significant because it tends to cause severe pain and neurological dysfunction due to its anatomical features.

Two surgical treatments for foraminal stenosis have been reported: spinal fusion [5–9] and foraminoplasty. Of these, fusion surgery seems to be the gold standard. The other method is minimally invasive full-endoscopic lumbar foraminoplasty (FELF) without fusion [10–13], which is a modification of transforaminal full-endoscopic discectomy [14–18]. It is possible to perform FELF under local anesthesia, which would be beneficial for high-risk patients, in particular the elderly and

K. Yamashita (✉)
Department of Orthopedics, Tokushima University School of Medicine, Tokushima, Japan

K. Sairyo (ed.), *Transforaminal Full-Endoscopic Lumbar Surgery Under the Local Anesthesia*, https://doi.org/10.1007/978-981-15-7023-0_9

those with significant comorbid conditions. The procedure is performed through an 8 mm skin incision and damage to the paravertebral muscles is minimal; this full-endoscopic technique is thus the least invasive lumbar surgery available at this time.

In the literature, we describe the indication, preoperative preparation, and surgical technique of FELF in detail.

9.1 Indication

There are several causes of lumbar foraminal stenosis, limbus vertebral fractures, degenerative spondylolisthesis, degenerative scoliosis, lumbar disc herniation in foramen, osteophyte of the superior articular process, and so on [19]. Best indications of FELF are lumbar disc herniation in foramen and osteophyte of the superior articular process. Basically, TE-LRD is available for all lumbar levels. Progressive spondylolisthesis and scoliosis are not good indication of FELF due to the possibility of further progression after FELF.

9.2 Preoperative Preparation

Lumbar foraminal stenosis could be easily diagnosed in para-sagittal MRI; however, selective nerve root block (SNRB) and CT scan are indispensable for the correct diagnosis of foraminal stenosis (Fig. 9.1). They show that the affected spinal nerve root is interrupted at foramen. Using MRI or CT scan, the surgeon should measure the insertion point and angle and then make their imagination of bone removing area (Fig. 9.2).

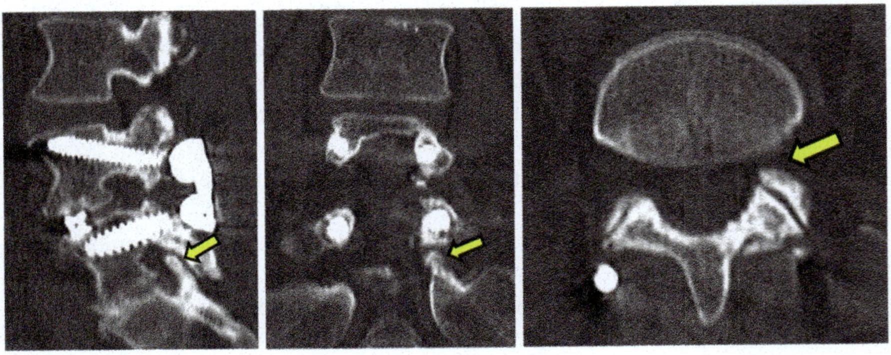

Fig. 9.1 CT scans before FELF. CT scans before full-endoscopic lumbar foraminoplasty. CT scans show left bony foraminal stenosis at the level of L5/S after L4/5 TLIF. There is an obvious protruding bone at the ventral aspect of upper articular process of the sacrum (arrow)

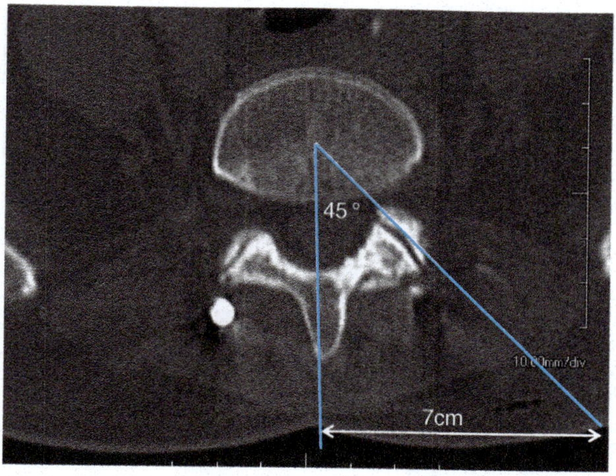

Fig. 9.2 Measurement of insertion point and angle. Using CT scan, appropriate distance from center line and angle can be measured. In this case, the insertion point is 7 cm from the center line and the insertion angle is 45°

9.3 Surgical Technique

The procedure should be performed under local anesthesia with the patient in the prone position on a radiolucent table. The skin entry point was about 6–8 cm from the midline. After administration of local anesthesia around the entry point, an 18-gauge spinal needle was inserted into the disc of concerned level, and an intra-operative discogram was obtained using a mixture of indigo carmine and contrast medium. Following insertion of a spinal needle into the disc under C-arm fluoroscopic guidance, a guide wire was inserted through the spinal needle, after which the needle was removed. An 8 mm skin incision was made and the tapered cannulated obturator was inserted along with a cannula into the foraminal area. The endoscope was then inserted into the foraminal space through the cannula. The ventral aspect of the superior articular process of the sacrum was removed carefully using a high-speed drill (Fig. 9.3a). Next, the blue-stained slightly bulging herniated nucleus pulposus (HNP) was exposed (Fig. 9.3b) and if needed, HNP was removed using small forceps and a radiofrequency wave system. Adequate decompression was achieved by careful removal of the residual ventral aspect of the superior articular process (Fig. 9.3c). The endoscope and cannula were then removed, which was followed by placement of a catheter, wound closure using a single stitch, and application of a sterile dressing. The procedure usually took under 60 min to perform and there was limited blood loss. Two hours after the surgery, the patient can stand up and walk without restriction. CT scans after FELF show the sufficient decompression of the left foramen (Fig. 9.4).

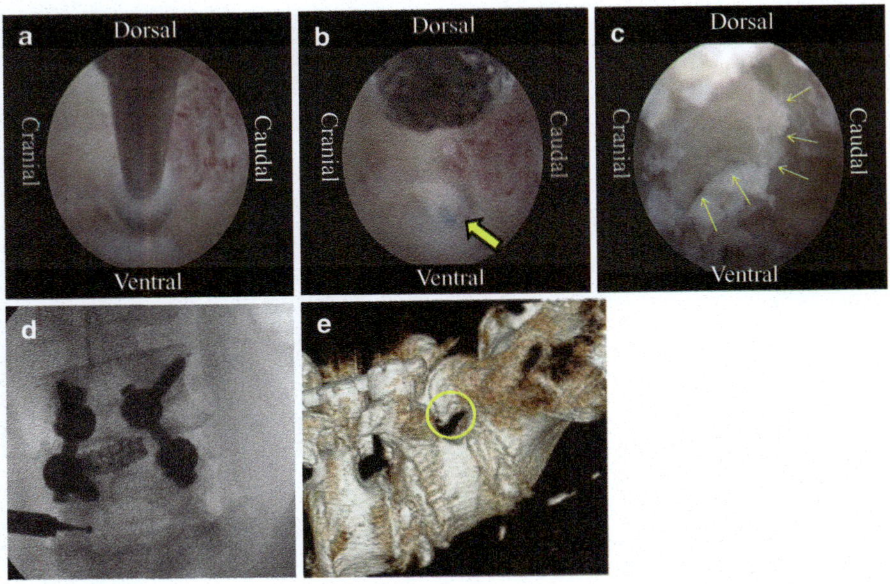

Fig. 9.3 The intraoperative endoscopic view. (**a**) The protruding bone was dug using a high-speed drill. (**b**) The blue stained nucleus pulposus was exposed (arrow). (**c**) The residual ventral aspect of the superior articular process (arrow) was broken off and removed. (**d**) The endoscopic procedure was done fluoroscopically. (**e**) The circle in the 3D-CT shows the field of endoscopic view

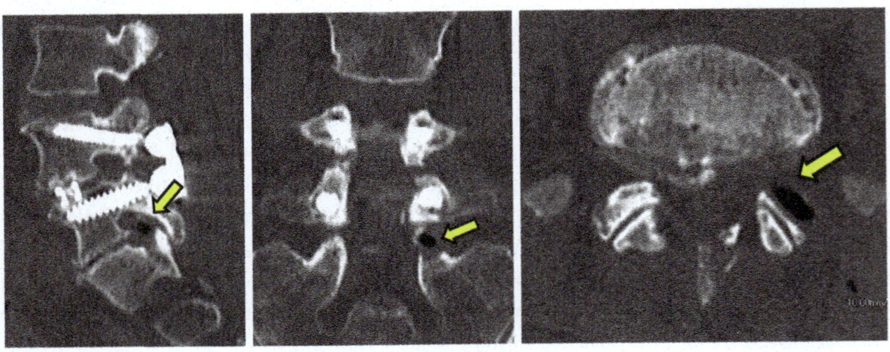

Fig. 9.4 CT scans after the PELF. The CT scans show sufficient decompression of the left foramen at L5/S (arrow)

9.4 Conclusion

FELF can be performed without fusion under local anesthesia and is performed through an 8 mm skin incision and damage to the paravertebral muscles is minimal, which is thus the least invasive lumbar surgery available for lumbar foraminal stenosis.

References

1. Putti V. New conceptions in the pathogenesis of sciatic pain. Lancet. 1927;2:53–60.
2. Mitchell C. Lumbosacral facetectomy for relief of sciatic pain. J Bone Joint Surg Br. 1934;36-B:230–7.
3. Arnoldi CC, Brodsky AE, Cauchoix J, Crock HV, Dommisse GF, Edgar MA, Gargano FP, Jacobson RE, Kirkaldy-Willis WH, Kurihara A, Langenskiold A, Macnab I, McIvor GW, Newman PH, Paine KW, Russin LA, Sheldon J, Tile M, Urist MR, Wilson WE, Wiltse LL. Lumbar spinal stenosis and nerve root entrapment syndromes. Definition and classification. Clin Orthop Relat Res. 1976;115:4–5.
4. Burton CV, Kirkaldy-Willis WH, Yong-Hing K, Heithoff KB. Causes of failure of surgery on the lumbar spine. Clin Orthop Relat Res. 1981;157:191–9.
5. Orita S, Yamagata M, Ikeda Y, Nakajima F, Aoki Y, Nakamura J, Takahashi K, Suzuki T, Ohtori S. Retrospective exploration of risk factors for L5 radiculopathy following lumbar floating fusion surgery. J Orthop Surg Res. 2015;10:164.
6. Alimi M, Hofstetter CP, Tsiouris AJ, Elowitz E, Härtl R. Extreme lateral interbody fusion for unilateral symptomatic vertical foraminal stenosis. Eur Spine J. 2015;24(3):346–52.
7. Jenis LG, An HS, Gordin R. Foraminal stenosis of the lumbar spine: a review of 65 surgical cases. Am J Orthop (Belle Mead NJ). 2001;30(3):205–11.
8. Merckaert S, Pierzchala K, Kulik G, Schizas C. Influence of anatomical variations on lumbar foraminal stenosis pathogenesis. Eur Spine J. 2015;24(2):313–8.
9. Lin JH, Chiang YH. Unilateral approach for bilateral foramen decompression in minimally invasive transforaminal interbody fusion. World Neurosurg. 2014;82(5):891–6.
10. Yeung A, Gore S. Endoscopic foraminal decompression for failed back surgery syndrome under local anesthesia. Int J Spine Surg. 2014;8 https://doi.org/10.14444/1022. eCollection.
11. Ahn Y, Oh HK, Kim H, Lee SH, Lee HN. Percutaneous endoscopic lumbar foraminotomy: an advanced surgical technique and clinical outcomes. Neurosurgery. 2014;75(2):124–33.
12. Ruetten S, Komp M, Merk H, Godolias G. Use of newly developed instruments and endoscopes: full-endoscopic resection of lumbar disc herniations via the interlaminar and lateral transforaminal approach. J Neurosurg Spine. 2007;6(6):521–30.
13. Henmi T, Terai T, Hibino N, Yoshioka S, Kondo K, Goda Y. Percutaneous endoscopic lumbar discectomy utilizing ventral epiduroscopic observation technique and foraminoplasty for transligamentous extruded nucleus pulposus: technical note. J Neurosurg Spine. 2015;13:1–6.
14. Yeung AT. The evolution of percutaneous spinal endoscopy and discectomy: state of the art. Mt Sinai J Med. 2000;67:327–32.
15. Yeung AT, Tsou PM. Posterolateral endoscopic excision for lumbar disc herniation: surgical technique, outcome, and complications in 307 consecutive cases. Spine. 2002;27:722–31.
16. Yeung AT, Yeung CA. Minimally invasive techniques for the management of lumbar disc herniation. Orthop Clin North Am. 2007;38(3):363–72.
17. Sairyo K, Egawa H, Matsuura T, Takahashi M, Higashino K, Sakai T, Suzue N, Hamada D, Goto T, Takata Y, Nishisho T, Goda Y, Sato R, Tsutsui T, Tonogai I, Kondo K, Tezuka F, Mineta K, Sugiura K, Takeuchi M, Dezawa A. State of the art: transforaminal approach for percutaneous endoscopic lumbar discectomy under local anesthesia. J Med Investig. 2014;61(3–4):217–25.
18. Sairyo K, Nagamachi A. State-of-the-art management of low back pain in athletes: instructional lecture. J Orthop Sci. 2016;21(3):263–72.
19. Epstein NE. Foraminal and far lateral lumbar disc herniations: surgical alternatives and outcome measures. Spinal Cord. 2002;40(10):491–500.

10 Full-Endoscopic Lateral Recess Decompression (Ventral Facetectomy)

Kazuta Yamashita

Abstract

There are three types of LSS, intervertebral foraminal stenosis, lateral recess stenosis, and central canal stenosis. Using the minimally invasive new endoscopic technique, transforaminal full-endoscopic lateral recess decompression (TE-LRD), both foraminal and lateral recess stenosis can be decompressed. We named full-endoscopic venrtral facetectomy (Sairyo et al., J Orthop Sci 23(2):229–36, 2018). TE-LRD should have benefits in elderly patients with LSS and poor general condition due to multiple comorbidities because it can be performed under local anesthesia. In this chapter, we describe this new technique in detail.

Full-endoscopic surgery for the lumbar spine, which was established in the last decade, requires only an 8-mm skin incision and causes minimal damage to the paravertebral muscles; thus, it is considered to be a minimally invasive technique for spinal surgery. In this decade, full-endoscopic discectomy techniques have been applied for lumbar spinal stenosis (LSS), the transforaminal (TF) method for foraminal stenosis under local anesthesia, and the interlaminar (IL) method for central and lateral recess stenosis under general anesthesia. In this chapter, we describe simultaneous decompression of the lateral recess and foraminal stenosis using the TF approach. Using this technique, which is called transforaminal full-endoscopic lateral recess decompression (TE-LRD), both foraminal and lateral recess stenosis can be decompressed [1–3]. TE-LRD should have benefits in elderly patients with LSS and poor general condition due to multiple comorbidities because it can be performed under local anesthesia.

K. Yamashita (✉)
Department of Orthopedics, Tokushima University School of Medicine, Tokushima, Japan

K. Sairyo (ed.), *Transforaminal Full-Endoscopic Lumbar Surgery Under the Local Anesthesia*, https://doi.org/10.1007/978-981-15-7023-0_10

10.1 Indication

There are three types of LSS: intervertebral foraminal stenosis, lateral recess stenosis, and central canal stenosis [4]. As mentioned in Chap. 9, intervertebral foraminal stenosis can be treated using the full-endoscopic lumbar foraminoplasty (FELF) technique. The best indication of TE-LRD is unilateral recess stenosis attending with disc herniation. On the other hand, central canal stenosis with thick flavum is a poor indication for this technique. Normally, total removal of the thick flavum is difficult using this technique because of its insertion angle. Partial removal of thick flavum is not enough for remission. And also, progressive spondylolisthesis and scoliosis are not a good indication of TE-LRD due to the possibility of further progression after this technique. Although TE-LRD is available for all lumbar levels, we had sometimes encountered difficult L5/S1 cases with high iliac case.

10.2 Preoperative Preparation

Lumbar lateral recess stenosis could be diagnosed using axial MRI and CT myelogram (Fig. 10.1). Using these image findings, the surgeon should measure the insertion point and angle and make imagination of bone removing area in the same manner of FELF described in Chap. 9 (Fig. 10.1b).

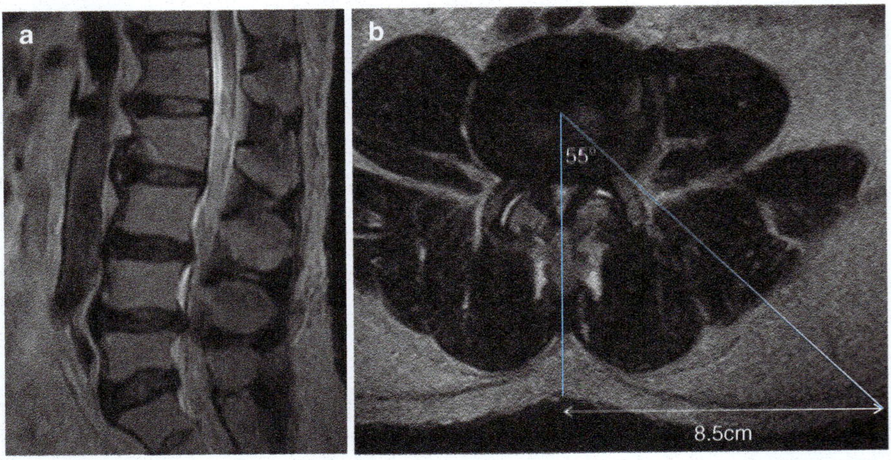

Fig. 10.1 Preoperative MRI measurement of insertion distance and angle. MRI before TE-LRD show bilateral recess stenosis at the level of L4/5 (**a**, **b**). Using axial MRI, appropriate distance from center line and angle can be measured. In this case, insertion point is 8.5 cm from center line and insertion angle is 55°

10.3 Surgical Technique

This is an advanced technique of FELF as described in Chap. 9. After widening the intervertebral foramen using the FELF technique, the cannula is further proceeded into the spinal canal. TE-LRD requires further removal of SAP. We usually start SAP drilling from the lateral side of the SAP, and then move the cannula to the tip of the SAP. Further drilling of the SAP should be done from the tip to pedicle. During this drilling using a surgical bur, we changed hand position to downwards gradually (hand-down technique) (Fig. 10.2) so that the lateral recess can be decompressed; it means that the facet joint space and flavum would be exposed (Fig. 10.3a). The SAP was drilled and shaved completely, so that both foraminal and lateral

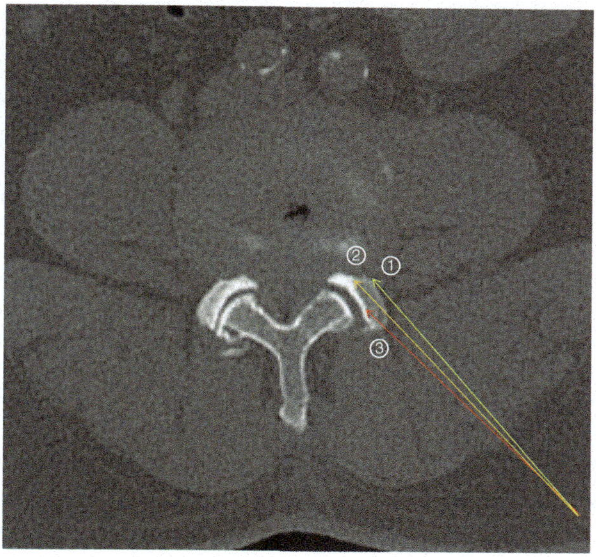

Fig. 10.2 Preoperative axial CT and plan of drilling angle (hand down technique). Using CT scan, surgeon can get a plan of SAP drilling. First, cannula should be set just lateral side of SAP and SAP drilling should be done from lateral to medial with changing hand position downwards (① → ② → ③)

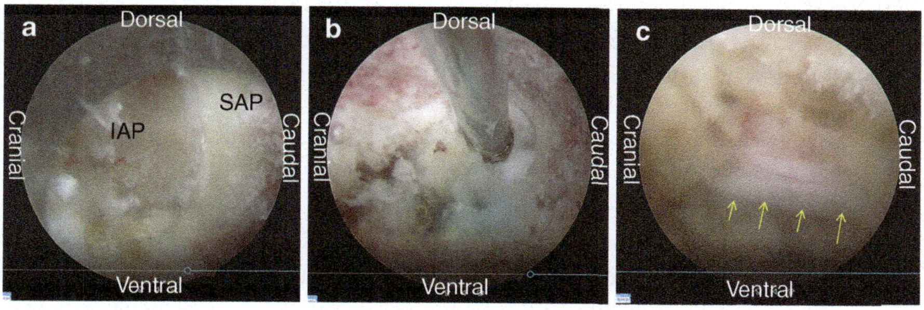

Fig. 10.3 The intraoperative endoscopic view. (**a**) Using high-speed drill, facet joint space and flavum was exposed. *IAP* inferior articular process, *SAP* superior articular process. (**b**) After drilling of SAP, flavum and blue stained nucleus pulposus was exposed. Red color is pedicle. (**c**) After complete removal of SAP and partial resection of flavum, the lateral wall of the traversing nerve root is exposed (arrows)

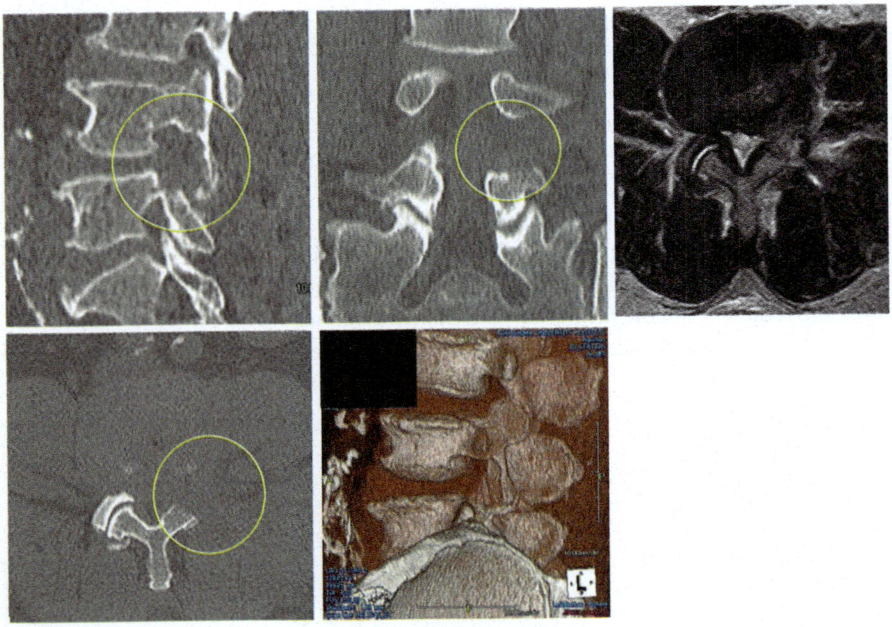

Fig. 10.4 CT scans and axial MRI after the TE-LRD. The CT scans and MRI show the sufficient decompression of the left foramen and lateral recess of L4/5 (circles)

recess decompression could be performed endoscopically at the same time (Fig. 10.3b). The completely decompressed traversing nerve root is clearly visible just around the pedicle (Fig. 10.3c). The lateral wall of the traversing nerve root is completely resected. The procedure usually took under 80 min to perform and there was limited blood loss. One drain tube should be inserted via cannula for prevention of postoperative hematoma. Two hours after the surgery, the patient can stand up and walk without restriction. As shown in Fig. 10.4, the ventral side of the facet joint is removed with enlargement of the lateral recess; thus, this procedure is also called full-endoscopic lumbar ventral facetectomy (FEVF). With this technique, the lateral recess stenosis as well as the foraminal stenosis can be decompressed simultaneously under local anesthesia.

10.4 Conclusion

TE-LRD/venteral facetectomy would be at present considered a minimally invasive technique on the basis of the damage to the spinal structures including back muscles as well as the method of anesthesia for the surgeries. Using this technique, both foraminal and lateral recess stenosis can be decompressed. In progressing aging society, surgery in local anesthesia would be minimally invasive for the elderly people compared to general anesthesia.

References

1. Sairyo K, Chikawa T, Nagamachi A. State-of-the-art transforaminal percutaneous endoscopic lumbar surgery under local anesthesia: discectomy, foraminoplasty, and ventral facetectomy. J Orthop Sci. 2018;23(2):229–36.
2. Kapetanakis S, Gkantsinikoudis N, Papathanasiou JV, Charitoudis G, Thomaidis T. Percutaneous endoscopic ventral facetectomy: an innovative substitute of open decompression surgery for lateral recess stenosis surgical treatment? J Craniovertebr Junction Spine. 2018;9(3):188–95.
3. Lewandrowski KU. Readmissions after outpatient transforaminal decompression for lumbar foraminal and lateral recess stenosis. Int J Spine Surg. 2018;12(3):342–51.
4. Steurer J, Roner S, Gnannt R, Hodler J. Quantitative radiologic criteria for the diagnosis of lumbar spinal stenosis: a systematic literature review. BMC Musculoskelet Disord. 2011;12:175.

Part IV

Thermal Annuloplasty (Full-endo TA)

Indication and High-Intensity Zone (HIZ) 11

Yoichiro Takata

Abstract

High-intensity zone (HIZ) is located in the posterior annulus fibrosus of the intervertebral disc on the T2-weighted lumbar magnetic resonance (MR) images. HIZ is described as an indicator of internal disc disruption or tear of annulus fibrosus. Discogenic low back pain (DLBP) with HIZ can be diagnosed with the MR image findings of HIZ in the target disc, provocative discography, and leakage of contrast medium into the fissure of annular tear. DLBP with HIZ can be treated by full-endo thermal annuloplasty (TA) under local anesthesia. The indication of full-endo TA for DLBP is the cases unresponsive to conservative treatment and concordant LBP during discography to the target disc.

Keywords

High-intensity zone · Magnetic resonance images · Discography

11.1 Background

The intervertebral disc has a multilayered structure that consists of a nucleus pulposus, an annulus fibrosus with nerve fibers only on the surface, and two cartilage endplates that cover the upper and lower surfaces of vertebral bodies. The main function of the intervertebral disc is transmitting the load and providing the flexibility to the spine.

As disc degeneration develops with aging, there is ingrowth of nerve fibers, including nociceptive fibers (sensory neurons that respond to noxious stimuli) and

Y. Takata (✉)
Department of Orthopedics, Tokushima University, Tokushima, Japan
e-mail: yoichiro76@tokushima-u.ac.jp

K. Sairyo (ed.), *Transforaminal Full-Endoscopic Lumbar Surgery Under the Local Anesthesia*, https://doi.org/10.1007/978-981-15-7023-0_11

vascular granulation tissue deeper into the annulus fibrosus [1] resulting in discogenic low back pain (DLBP).

The treatment of DLBP is basically conservative treatment. Surgical treatment is considered for patients unresponsive to conservative treatment. Surgical treatments include disc excision with laminectomy, spinal fusion, and artificial disc replacement. However, such surgical treatments need general anesthesia, large skin incision, and loss of normal spinal mobility and require long recovery time. Minimally invasive procedures have many benefits such as small skin incision, less blood loss, less invasive to paravertebral muscle, lower risk of postoperative infection, and faster recovery time.

11.2 Definition of HIZ

High-intensity zone (HIZ) was first reported by Aprill and Bogduk in 1992 as a high signal intensity area located in the substance of annulus fibrosus on T2-weighted magnetic resonance (MR) images of lumbar spine (Fig. 11.1). HIZ is described as an indicator of internal disc disruption or tear of annulus fibrosus. Originally, HIZ was defined as a high-intensity signal on T2-weighted MR images, located posteriorly in the annulus fibrosus, which is clearly dissociated from the signal of the nucleus pulposus, which was surrounded by a low-intensity signal of the annulus fibrosus and in turn was appreciably brighter than the cerebrospinal fluid signal at the same level.

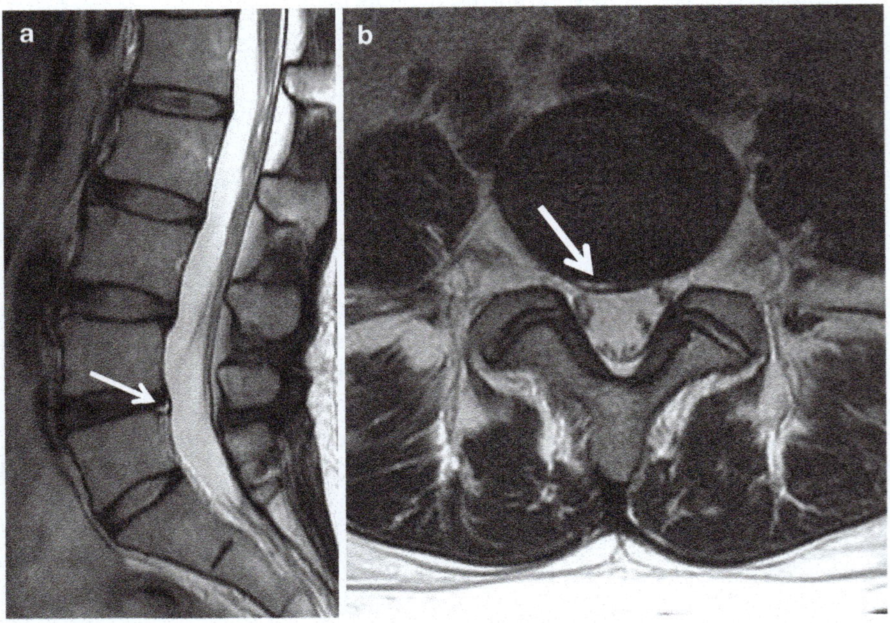

Fig. 11.1 Magnetic resonance (MR) images showing high-intensity signal in the posterior annulus fibrosus on sagittal (**a**) and axial (**b**) on T2-weighted image (white arrow)

11.2.1 Prevalence of HIZ

The prevalence of HIZs ranges from 28% to 59% in patients with LBP; alternatively its prevalence has also been reported to be 3.2–56% in asymptomatic patients [2–9]. A prospective observation study of patients with LBP showed that 59% had HIZ-positive LBP and 24% of HIZ-positive had no LBP [2].

11.2.2 Location of HIZ

HIZs occur mainly at the posterior part of the annulus fibrosus; however, some recent reports indicated that a similar lesion occurring at the posterolateral annulus fibrosus should also be considered as HIZ [6, 10–12]. Another study reported that HIZ appeared in the anterior part of annulus fibrosus in 42.4% in a large population study [13]. They also classified signal intensity change of HIZ on T1-weighted MR image into three types (low, high, and iso-intensity). HIZ with T1W iso-intensity type was most prevalent (71.8%), followed by T1W high intensity (21.4%) and T1W low intensity (6.8%). More than two-thirds of HIZs are identified at lower lumbar segments (L4/5 and L5/S) [7, 10–12]. The prevalence of multi-level HIZs was 16.5% [12], and 75% of cases with multi-level HIZs exhibited HIZs in an adjacent disc.

11.2.3 Pathology of HIZ

Histological findings of HIZ showed the formation of vascularized granulation tissue in the outer region of the annulus fibrosus. Immunohistochemical analysis showed that an abundance of tumor necrosis factor-alpha-positive cells and some CD68-positive cells were observed in the HIZ [14].

11.2.4 Natural History of HIZ

The follow-up study of the patients with HIZ showed that HIZs were found to have resolved in 26.6%, improved in 14%, worsened in 18.8%, and remained unchanged in 40.6% in 1–4 years. Among the subjects with improvement of LBP, 25% showed resolution of HIZ, 50% unchanged, and the rest became worse. No significant correlation was observed between the HIZ changes and subjective symptoms [9].

11.3 Diagnosis of DLBP with HIZ

A precise diagnosis is important when treating DLBP. The characteristic symptom of DLBP is typically pain in forward bending, not in backward bending, and improvement with recumbency. No specific features of symptom make the diagnosis of DLBP difficult.

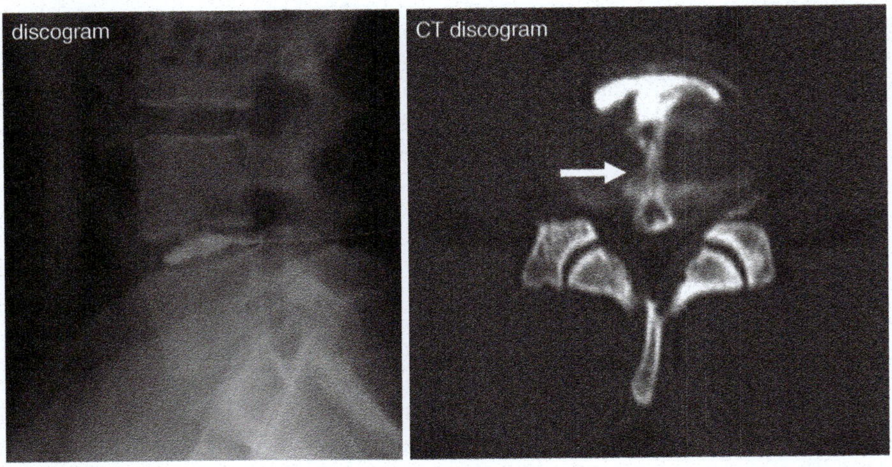

Fig. 11.2 Discogram and CT discogram showing leakage of contrast medium through the fissure of posterior annulus fibrosus, which is called toxic/ painful annular tear (white arrow)

MR images and discography are the most important modalities to diagnose DLBP. Discographic findings showing the leakage of contrast medium into the epidural space through annular tear are the most important findings to diagnose DLBP with HIZ (Fig. 11.2). Studies have demonstrated that in morphologically abnormal discs, a significant correlation exists between HIZ-positive discs and exact or concordant LBP on provocative discography. If HIZs exist at multi-levels, provocative discographies to each disc level should be conducted to clarify the responsible intervertebral disc level.

11.4 Thermal Annuloplasty

Various minimally invasive procedures for the treatment of DLBP, such as intradiscal electrothermal therapy (IDET), intradiscal injection, and full-endoscopic thermal annuloplasty (Full-endo TA), have been reported. Full-endo TA was first reported by Tsou et al. [15] as the surgical technique using posterior transforaminal selective endoscopic discectomy to treat chronic DLBP. Full-endo TA is minimally invasive and can be performed under local anesthesia via an 8 mm skin incision, and it provides the advantage of direct visualization of the degenerated disc and annular tear by means of a spinal endoscope. The most important difference between IDET and full-endo TA is direct observation of degenerated or ruptured annulus fibrosus. Full-endoscopic surgery routinely uses indigo carmine, a blue color dye, for intradiscal staining. Indigo carmine selectively stains the more acidic and fragmented degenerated nucleus pulposus, as demonstrated by direct visualization. Under endoscopic visualization, radiofrequency (RF) electrode is introduced into the annular fissure, already marked by indigo carmine. A degenerated nucleus pulposus will be also stained by indigo carmine and can be removed by rongeurs. The HIZ site can

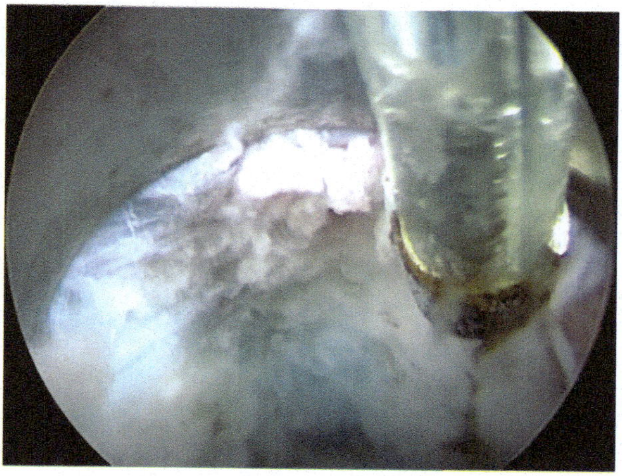

Fig. 11.3 Endoscopic view showing ablation of red nucleus pulposus suggesting inflammation and/or new vessels penetrating the mass with radiofrequency bipolar coagulator

be ablated with a radiofrequency coagulator with alternating current (1.7–4.0 MHz) using Trigger-Flex® bipolar coagulator (Fig. 11.3).

11.5 Indications

The indications of TA for DLBP are repetitive chronic LBP, failure of conservative treatment, provocative pain, and temporary pain relief on discography to the target disc. If injection of contrast medium into the disc space triggers concordant strong pain, the intervertebral disc is considered to be the pain source. Full-endo TA is effective in the case of center protrusion type of herniation with HIZ [16].

As full-endo TA uses the same approach with transforaminal FED, all cases who can be treated by transforaminal approach will be indicated.

11.6 Contraindications

Patients with aggressive disc degeneration, disc collapse, and symptomatic paralysis should not be the indication of full-endo TA. Spinal deformity with instability, infection, and tumor cases are not the candidates for full-endo TA. Severe collapse of the intervertebral disc space makes it difficult to insert the endoscope without endplate injury. Spinal canal stenosis with paralysis or radiculopathy should be treated by open laminectomy under general anesthesia. Migrated herniated nucleus pulposus (HNP) cannot be treated only by TA technique.

References

1. Coppes MH, Marani E, Thomeer RT, Groen GJ. Innervation of "painful" lumbar discs. Spine (Phila Pa 1976). 1997;22(20):2342–9.

2. Carragee EJ, Paragioudakis SJ, Khurana S. Volvo Award winner in clinical studies: lumbar high-intensity zone and discography in subjects without low back problems. Spine (Phila Pa 1976). 2000;25:2987.
3. Ricketson R, Simmons JW, Hauser BO. The prolapsed intervertebral disc. The high-intensity zone with discography correlation. Spine (Phila Pa 1976). 1997;21(23):2758–62.
4. Park K-W, Song K-S, Chung JY, Choi J-M, Lee J-H, Lee C-K, et al. High-intensity zone on L-spine MRI: clinical relevance and association with trauma history. Asian Spine J. 2007;1(1):38–42.
5. Takatalo J, Karppinen J, Niinimaki J, Taimela S, Mutanen P, Sequeiros RB, et al. Association of modic changes, Schmorl's nodes, spondylolytic defects, high-intensity zone lesions, disc herniations, and radial tears with low back symptom severity among young Finnish adults. Spine (Phila Pa 1976). 2012;37:1231–9.
6. Liu C, Cai H-X, Zhang J-F, Ma J-J, Lu Y-J, Fan S-W. Quantitative estimation of the high-intensity zone in the lumbar spine: comparison between the symptomatic and asymptomatic population. Spine J. 2014;14:391–6.
7. Lam KS, Carlin D, Mulholland RC. Lumbar disc high-intensity zone: the value and significance of provocative discography in the determination of the discogenic pain source. Eur Spine J. 2000;9(1):36–41.
8. Rankine JJ, Gill KP, Hutchinson CE, Ross ER, Williamson JB. The clinical significance of the high-intensity zone on lumbar spine magnetic resonance imaging. Spine (Phila Pa 1976). 1999;24(18):1913.
9. Mitra D, Cassar-Pullicino VN, McCall IW. Longitudinal study of high intensity zones on MR of lumbar intervertebral discs. Clin Radiol. 2004;59(11):1002–8.
10. Saifuddin A, Braithwaite I, White J, Taylor BA, Renton P. The value of lumbar spine magnetic resonance imaging in the demonstration of anular tears. Spine (Phila Pa 1976). 1998;23(4):453–7.
11. Schellhas KP, Pollei SR, Gundry CR, Heithoff KB. Lumbar disc high-intensity zone. Correlation of magnetic resonance imaging and discography. Spine (Phila Pa 1976). 1996;21(1):79–86.
12. Wang Z-X, Hu Y-G. High-intensity zone (HIZ) of lumbar intervertebral disc on T2-weighted magnetic resonance images: spatial distribution, and correlation of distribution with low back pain (LBP). Eur Spine J. 2012;21(7):1311–5.
13. Teraguchi M, Samartzis D, Hashizume H, Yamada H, Muraki S, Oka H, et al. Classification of high intensity zones of the lumbar spine and their association with other spinal MRI phenotypes: the Wakayama spine study. PLoS One. 2016;11:1–15.
14. Dongfeng R, Hou S, Wu W, Wang H, Shang W, Tang J, et al. The expression of tumor necrosis factor-α and CD68 in high-intensity zone of lumbar intervertebral disc on magnetic resonance image in the patients with low back pain. Spine (Phila Pa 1976). 2011;36(6):E429–33.
15. Tsou PM, Yeung CA, Yeung AT. Posterolateral transforaminal selective endoscopic discectomy and thermal annuloplasty for chronic lumbar discogenic pain: a minimal access visualized intradiscal surgical procedure. Spine J. 2004;4:564–73.
16. Ahn Y, Lee S-H. Outcome predictors of percutaneous endoscopic lumbar discectomy and thermal annuloplasty for discogenic low back pain. Acta Neurochir. 2010;152:1695–702.

Full-Endoscopic Thermal Annuloplasty for Athletes

12

Hiroaki Manabe

Abstract

Many athletes who repeatedly load the spine suffer from back pain. Although conservative therapy is the first choice, surgery may be the option in cases such as opposing conservative therapy or aiming for an early return. Athletes should be treated as minimally invasive as possible. Full-endoscopic surgery is one of the minimally invasive surgeries in current low back pain surgery. Recently, Full-endoscopic discectomy (FED) combined with thermal annuloplasty (TA) for discogenic pain is taking place. FED/TA has the advantage of allowing direct visualization of degenerative intervertebral discs and annular tears under endoscopy and providing access to the intervertebral disc without damaging the back muscles, which can be performed safely and accurately. For the reason, FED/TA is useful for elite athletes to enable early return to competition sports. In this chapter, we report the usefulness of FED/TA in elite athletes with discogenic low back pain.

Keywords

Low back pain · Full-endoscopic surgery · Thermal annuloplasty · Elite athletes

12.1 Introduction

Many elite athletes experience back pain at least once during a sports career, and back pain is a serious problem that requires early diagnosis and appropriate treatment. Among them, pain caused by the intervertebral disc is relatively common,

H. Manabe (✉)
Department of Orthopedics, Tokushima University, Tokushima, Japan

K. Sairyo (ed.), *Transforaminal Full-Endoscopic Lumbar Surgery Under the Local Anesthesia*, https://doi.org/10.1007/978-981-15-7023-0_12

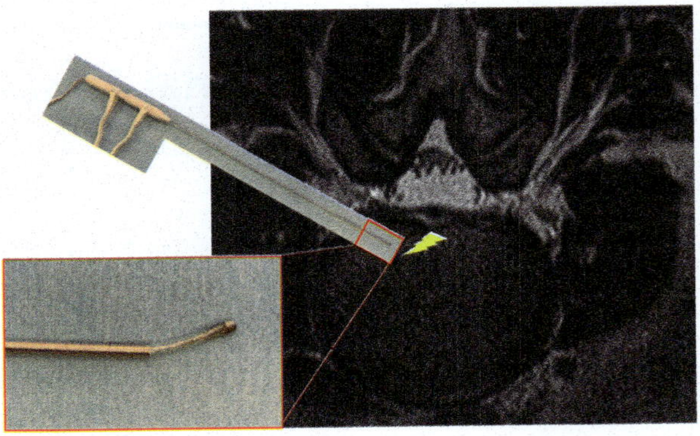

Fig. 12.1 Panel shows a bipolar probe coagulating a damaged annulus in which a high signal intensity zone and a painful annular tear are causing low back pain

suggesting that it accounts for up to 26–42% of all cases of back pain [1–3]. Low back pain is often treated conservatively, but surgery may be indicated if the pain is refractory to conservative treatment or if it is desired to return to early play. In the case of athlete surgery, it is desirable that the treatment be minimally invasive.

Full-endoscopic discectomy (FED), developed by Yeung and Tsou [4], is one of the least invasive treatments available for back pain and is becoming increasingly popular. FED is generally performed via a transforaminal approach under local anesthesia and requires an 8 mm skin incision. It is minimally invasive and protects the back muscles [5, 6]. The FED technique is also used for chronic intervertebral back pain [7, 8]. After selective discectomy of the degenerative disc, the annular tear are cauterized by thermal annuloplasty (TA) using a bipolar (Fig. 12.1). This procedure (FED/TA) has been reported to be an effective treatment for discogenic pain [9].

This chapter describes FED/TA strategies for athletes and reports on cases of elite athletes with back pain that were properly treated with FED/TA.

12.2 Indication

12.2.1 Discogenic Pain

In some cases, typical findings such as high intensity zone (HIZ) are not confirmed on the image, sufficient preoperative examination is required for a definitive diagnosis.

12.3 Diagnosis

Discogenic pain is sometimes treated as an unexplained back pain because there are some cases in which diagnosis is difficult based on physical and image findings alone. Unlike the disc herniation, there is no characteristic of lower limbs as a characteristic physical finding. In a typical case, low back pain is caused by increasing the load on the intervertebral disc at the time of forward flexion. HIZ is an important finding that reflects the secondary inflammatory changes that accumulate in the anterior annulus [10] and is displayed in the posterior annulus with high intensity changes on MRI T2-weighted images. Discography and discoblock are indispensable for a definitive diagnosis, and a diagnosis of discogenic pain is made by confirming the pain reproduction due to discography and the subsequent disappearance of pain due to discoblock.

12.4 Preoperative Preparation

Preoperative discography and CT imaging in the prone position can determine the appropriate puncture point expected during the operation. In addition, the site of the contrast medium leakage and/or HIZ should be carefully confirmed by discography CT and/or MRI, and corresponded to the plain radiograph.

12.5 Surgical Technique

12.5.1 Insertion Position

Although there are several approaches to the FED method, this method uses the transforaminal approach. In addition to being able to reach the intervertebral disc with minimal invasion of the paraspinal muscles, it can directly and pinpointly treat HIZ and annular tear. Furthermore, since it can be performed under local anesthesia, performed on patients with poor general condition. Although the insertion point depends on the pelvic height, it is often about 6–8 mm from the midline and advisable to record the insertion point during the discography performed before surgery. The skin incision should be 8 mm, which is the width of the endoscope, but the transversal incision has the advantage that the wound is not conspicuous and the endoscope can be easily controlled.

12.5.2 Endoscope

If there is no complication of disc herniation or foraminal stenosis, basically, the inside-out method is used. First, local anesthesia is performed with 1% lidocaine at the puncture site, and it is added to the fascia, muscle layer, and annulus fibrosus. Then, a 21 G needle, the diameter of which the guide wire passes, is inserted into the intervertebral disc from the Kambin's triangle zone, and it is confirmed through fluoroscopy that the tip is at the optimal position immediately below the lesion site. After that, 1% lidocaine and contrast medium mixed with indigo carmine are injected. At this time, low back pain may be induced by an increase in intervertebral disc pressure. A guide wire is inserted through the needle, and a serial dilator is sequentially installed to guide the cannula into the intervertebral disc after enlarging the invasion path. By applying local anesthesia to the annulus fibrosus, pain during insertion is reduced. If it is difficult to place the endoscope directly into the disc due to the stimulating of the exiting nerve root, performing the approach from the outside according to the outside-in method (described in another chapter), or expanding the intervertebral foramen with a drill, the range of motion of the nerve root is improved, and procedure is possible without stimulating the nerve root. Exiting nerve root stimulating pain can be avoided by shifting the incision inward, but it is difficult to reach the lesion site. In this procedure, it is important to reach the lesion site with a pinpoint, and should be understood that the arrival point differs considerably depending on the insertion angle. After placing the endoscope in the disc, the bird's-eye view confirms whether the posterior annulus is observable angle.

12.5.3 Resection of Degenerated Disc

After the endoscope is placed, nucleotomy is performed to remove degenerated discs. If the patient suddenly complains of pain during the procedure in the intervertebral disc, it is a sign that the lesion is close. In that case, it is necessary to remove the surrounding nucleus pulposus stained with indigo carmine little by little while cauterizing as appropriate. Excision of the surrounding soft tissue often reveals reddened painful annular tear (Fig. 12.2). If HIZ or painful annular tear is not clear during surgery [10], perform the procedure by comparing the endoscope position in the intraoperative fluoroscopic image with the contrast medium leaking site in the preoperative CT image. When confirming the site, it is easy to have an image that matches the lesion with the current treatment site by projecting the bipolar tip.

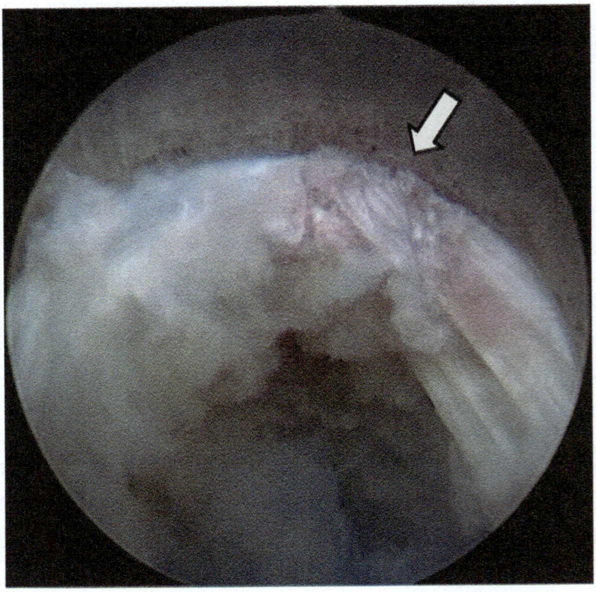

Fig. 12.2 Arrow indicates painful annulus tears with redness

12.5.4 Treatment of HIZ and Painful Annular Tear

When the redness area corresponding to HIZ is stimulated with a bipolar tip, the patient often complains of severe pain. In this case, cauterization is started around the reddened area, the procedure is gradually advanced to the center, and finally the entire lesion is cauterized and coagulated. In our hospital, radiofrequency bipolar ablation uses Trigger-Flex manufactured by elliquence (New York, USA), which is useful not only for cauterized and coagulated of lesions but also for hemostasis and transpiration of soft tissues. High-frequency radio waves are short waves of 2 MHz or higher and can be applied to the tissue at high density and intensively to reduce surrounding tissue damage. The ablated lesion does not cause stimulus pain, and we can judge the end point of operation.

12.5.5 Closure

The drain tube is placed in the intervertebral disc through a cannula, and the skin incision is sutured with absorbent thread and fixed with tape. The drain tube is removed the day after surgery.

12.5.6 Postoperative Therapy

Two hours after surgery, walking is allowed. Because of local anesthesia, the patient can perform daily activities immediately after surgery, and discharge after drain tube removal. For athletes, active stretch and trunk training started early after surgery, and full return to sports is 6–8 weeks after surgery.

12.6 Cases [9]

Twelve elite athletes (11 men, 1 woman; mean age 27.9 years) who underwent FED/TA under local anesthesia were retrospectively examined. Clinical data for these 12 patients (with 17 affected intervertebral discs), including type of sport played, average duration of low back pain, level of intervertebral disc affected, presence or absence of a high signal intensity zone (HIZ) on magnetic resonance imaging (MRI), and whether the patient returned to competitive play after FED/TA, were reviewed. All patients were diagnosed on the basis of clinical symptoms and findings on computed tomography (CT) and MRI. Discography was performed in all cases to confirm reproducible pain.

The most common sport played was baseball ($n = 8$), followed by cycling ($n = 2$), tennis ($n = 1$), and hammer throw ($n = 1$). Average duration of low back pain was 24.3 months. Intervertebral disc levels affected were L4/5 ($n = 11$) and L5/S1 ($n = 6$). A HIZ was observed in nine intervertebral discs (Table 12.1). Although two patients required additional surgery, all patients were able to return to their original

Table 12.1 Demographics and clinical characteristics of 12 elite athletes with discogenic pain

Sex	Age (years)	Sport	Duration of low back pain (months)	Level	HIZ
Male	20	Baseball	8	L5/S	–
Male	35	Baseball	10	L4/5	–
Male	32	Baseball	12	L4/5	+
Male	35	Baseball	12	L4/5	+
Male	28	Keirin	26	L4/5	–
Male	28	Tennis	36	L4/5	+
Female	30	Hammer throw	120	L4/5	+
Male	20	Road bike	6	L4/5	–
				L5/S	–
Male	20	Baseball	9	L4/5	+
				L5/S	+
Male	30	Baseball	14	L4/5	–
				L5/S	+
Male	23	Baseball	19	L4/5	–
				L5/S	+
Male	34	Baseball	20	L4/5	–
				L5/S	+

HIZ: high signal intensity zone

competitive level of play. Duration for the return to play was 2.8 months after surgery except the two revision cases.

In additional thermal annuloplasty cases, low back pain improved considerably after surgery, but mild pain inducted at the time of bending forward during the competition (road bike) remained. Follow-up MRI showed the bulging of disc persisted at operated level; the second operation performed 10 months later. In another case of revision surgery, hernia-related lower extremity pain disappeared and low back pain improved enough to return to competition (tennis) after the first surgery. However, because the patient had pain due to synovitis associated with the original spondylolysis, direct repair was performed at the retired timing.

12.6.1 Representative Case [9]: A 30-Year-Old Female Hammer Throw Player

The patient had a more than 10-year history of low back pain of unspecified cause that did not respond to conservative treatment. T2-weighted images on MRI revealed a HIZ at L4/5 (Fig. 12.3a). We confirmed reproducible pain by using discography and temporary pain relief by discoblock (Fig. 12.3b, c) [9], and performed FED/TA at L4/5 under local anesthesia. The procedure time was 51 min with minimal intraoperative blood loss. The low back pain disappeared immediately after the surgery. She started conditioning after surgery, resumed hammer throw after 8 weeks, and was able to return original competition level 4 months later.

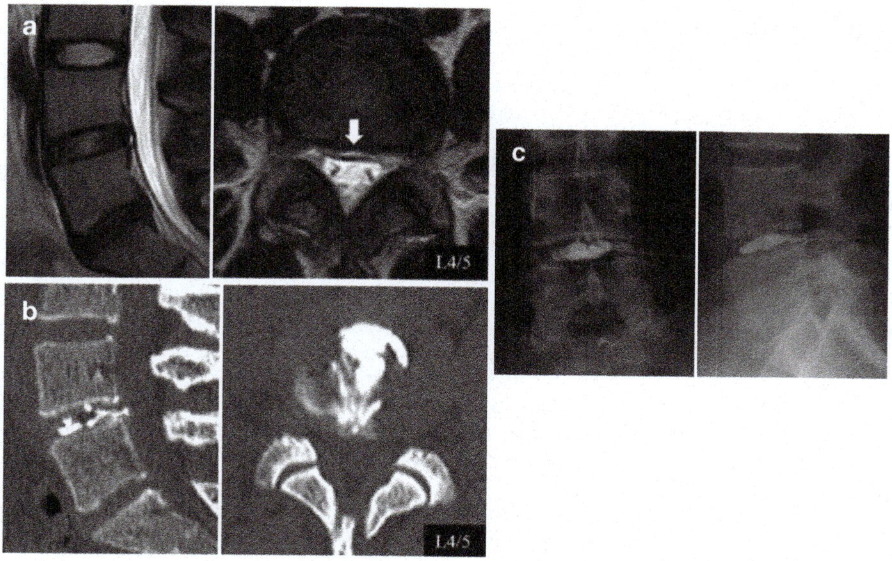

Fig. 12.3 (**a**) Sagittal and axial T2-weighted images showing a high signal intensity zone indicated by arrow at the level of L4/5 in a 30-year-old female hammer throw player. (**b**) Computed tomography images of discography showing that the contrast medium can be seen entering the posterior annulus where the high intensity signal zone is located. (**c**) Low back pain is confirmed to be reproducible by discography at L4–5

12.7 Conclusion

Although there are several surgical options for discogenic pain, curative surgery mainly consists of interbody fusion. However, radical surgery damages the back muscles and reduces lumbar mobility, making it unsuitable for athletes who want minimally invasive surgery. FED/TA was performed on 12 professional athletes with back pain due to the intervertebral disc and satisfactory results were obtained. This procedure is a reliable minimally invasive procedure for patients with discogenic pain. A variety of approaches can be used to perform FED, but the transforaminal approach is preferred because it allows access to the disc without damaging the back muscles, which is critical for elite athletes. In addition, FED/TA has the advantage of enabling direct visualization of degenerative discs and annular tear under endoscopy and treat them safely and accurately.

Conflicts of Interest and Source of Funding None declared.

Sources of support: None.

References

1. Schwarzer AC, Aprill CN, Derby R, Fortin J, Kine G, Bogduk N. The relative contributions of the disc and zygapophyseal joint in chronic low back pain. Spine. 1994;19:801–6.
2. DePalma MJ, Ketchum JM, Saullo T. What is the source of chronic low back pain and does age play a role? Pain Med. 2011;12:224–33.
3. Manchikanti L, Singh V, Pampati V, Damron KS, Barnhill RC, Beyer C, et al. Evaluation of the relative contributions of various structures in chronic low back pain. Pain Physician. 2001;4:308–16.
4. Yeung AT, Tsou PM. Posterolateral endoscopic excision for lumbar disc herniation: surgical technique, outcome, and complications in 307 consecutive cases. Spine. 2002;27:722–31.
5. Choi KC, Lee JH, Kim JS, Sabal LA, Lee S, Kim H, et al. Unsuccessful percutaneous endoscopic lumbar discectomy: a single-center experience of 10,228 cases. Neurosurgery. 2015;76:372–80.
6. Henmi T, Terai T, Hibino N, Yoshioka S, Kondo K, Goda Y, et al. Percutaneous endoscopic lumbar discectomy utilizing ventral epiduroscopic observation technique and foraminoplasty for transligamentous extruded nucleus pulposus: technical note. J Neurosurg Spine. 2016;24(2):275–80.
7. Tsou PM, Alan Yeung C, Yeung AT. Posterolateral transforaminal selective endoscopic discectomy and thermal annuloplasty for chronic lumbar discogenic pain: a minimal access visualized intradiscal surgical procedure. Spine J. 2004;4:564–73.
8. Sairyo K, Kitagawa Y, Dezawa A. Percutaneous endoscopic discectomy and thermal annuloplasty for professional athletes. Asian J Endosc Surg. 2013;6:292–7.
9. Manabe H, Yamashita K, Tezuka F, et al. Thermal annuloplasty using percutaneous endoscopic discectomy for elite athletes with discogenic low back pain. Neurol Med Chir (Tokyo). 2019;59:48–53.
10. Aprill C, Bogduk N. High-intensity zone: a diagnostic sign of painful lumbar disc on magnetic resonance imaging. Br J Radiol. 1992;65:361–9.

Part V
Others

13 Full-Endoscopic Trans-Kambin's Triangle Lumbar Interbody Fusion (Fullendo-KLIF)

Masatoshi Morimoto and Koichi Sairyo

Abstract

Full-endoscopic (fullendo) lumbar surgery was first introduced as a method for performing discectomy and has now been used for the decompression of lumbar spinal canal stenosis. Finally, the fullendo technique is started to be applied for lumbar interbody fusion (LIF). Since a cage has been inserted through Kambin triangle, it is called fullendo trans-Kambin triangle lumbar interbody fusion (KLIF). We created an original fullendo KLIF system. In this chapter, we explain the history of fullendo KLIF and introduce our technique.

Keywords

Fullendo KLIF · Kambin triangle · Interbody fusion · Full-endoscopic surgery

13.1 History of Fullendo KLIF

There are a variety of procedures for the lumbar interbody fusion (LIF) as shown in Fig. 13.1. The name was given anatomically such as anterior LIF (ALIF), lateral LIF (LLIF), trans-foraminal LIF (TLIF), and posterior LIF (PLIF). The lateral LIF has been further categorized in three types: oblique (OLIF), extreme lateral (XLIF), and direct lateral (DLIF).

Full-endoscopic (fullendo) lumbar surgery was first introduced as a method for performing discectomy and has now been used for the decompression of lumbar spinal canal stenosis. Finally, the fullendo technique is started to be appliedd for LIF. The basic concept is insertion of a cage through Kambin triangle in Fig. 13.2 under the guidance of the full endoscope.

M. Morimoto · K. Sairyo (✉)
Department of Orthopedics, Tokushima University, Tokushima, Japan

K. Sairyo (ed.), *Transforaminal Full-Endoscopic Lumbar Surgery Under the Local Anesthesia*, https://doi.org/10.1007/978-981-15-7023-0_13

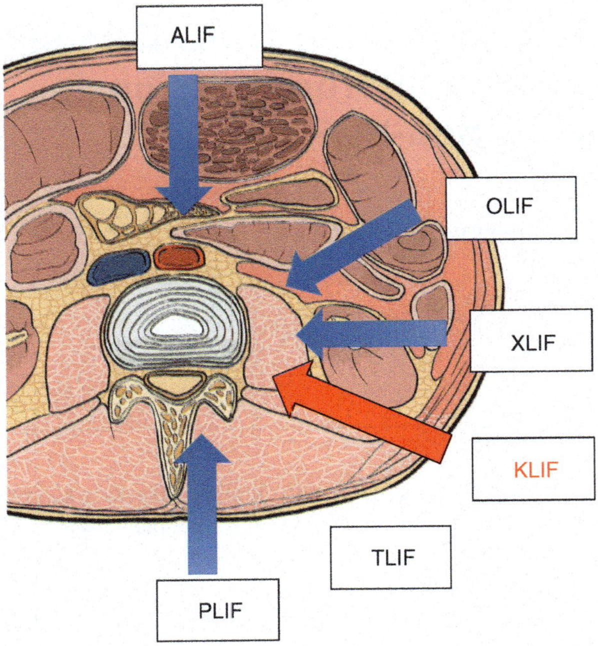

Fig. 13.1 Variety of procedures for the lumbar interbody fusion (LIF). The name is given anatomically such as anterior LIF (ALIF), lateral LIF (LLIF), trans-foraminal LIF (TLIF), and posterior LIF (PLIF). The lateral LIF is further categorized in three types: oblique (OLIF), extreme lateral (XLIF), and direct lateral (DLIF)

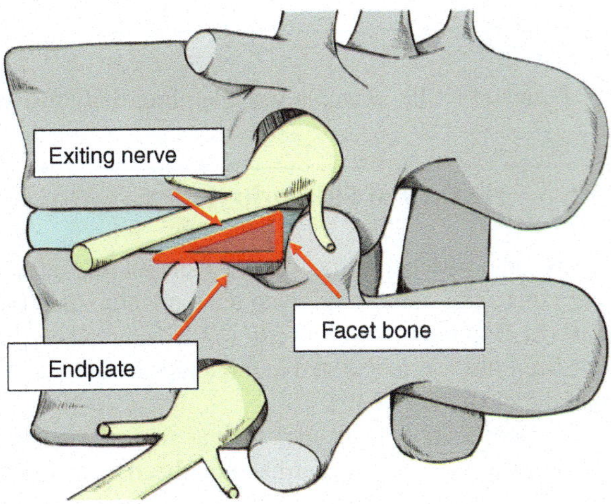

Fig. 13.2 Anatomical location of Kambin triangle. We propose that the technique to insert a cage through the Kambin triangle is trans-Kambin triangle LIF (KLIF)

In the literature, several doctors already reported their technique, and they named the technique as they like. So far, there is no consensus on the procedure being full-endoscopic insertion of a cage through Kambin triangle. For example, percutaneous endoscopic LIF [1] or full-endoscopic LIF [2] is reported, since LIF was performed using an endoscope. On the other hand, the procedure is similar to TLIF; thus, percutaneous endoscopic TLIF [3] or full-endoscopic TLIF [4] was proposed. However,

TLIF requires total facetectomy basically [5]. Fullendo trans-Kambin cage insertion does not need total facetectomy; thus, the technique would not be TLIF. Very recently, Lewandrowski et al. proposed lordotic endoscopic wedge lumbar interbody fusion (LEW-LIF) as the name for a similar technique [6].

All the techniques use a full-endoscope to create the route via which the cage is inserted, and the cage is inserted through Kambin triangle (Fig. 13.2). Hence, on anatomical grounds, we propose that this technique be named full-endoscopic trans-Kambin triangle LIF (fullendo-KLIF) [7].

13.2 Surgical Procedure

13.2.1 Surgical Indication

The best candidates for fullendo-KLIF at present are patients with a single-level disorder. Single-level fusion for conditions such as spondylolisthesis, scoliosis, discogenic pain, and Modic change, can now be treated using this procedure.

13.2.2 Surgical Technique

Prior to the fullendo-KLIF surgery, four percutaneous pedicle screws (PPS) are installed (Fig. 13.3), so that slippage reduction and disc height widening are conducted as much as possible. Then, the cannula of full endoscope is docked on the superior articular process (SAP). In Fig. 13.3, the radiograph indicates the location of PPSs and a cannula (left, Fig. 13.3). Figure 13.4 indicates the endoscopic view of the SAP. Usually, the bone surface of the SAP can be seen; however, in case the bone is covered with soft issue or capsule, KLIF starter is available (Fig. 13.5). The

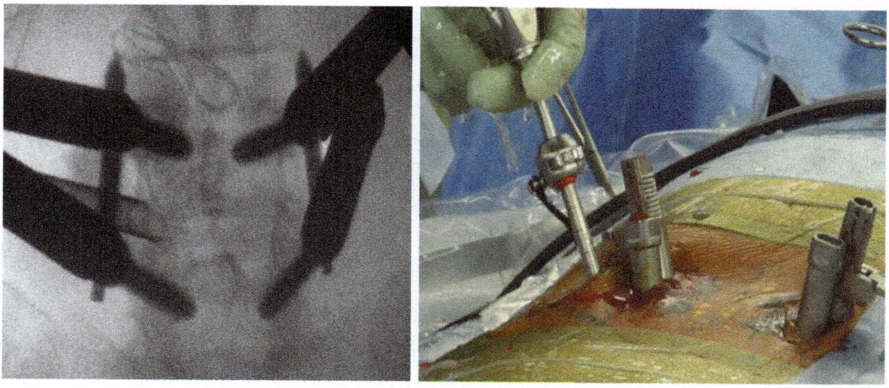

Fig. 13.3 Four percutaneous pedicle screws (PPS) and a cannula for the full endoscope installation. After installation of four PPSs, the cannula of full endoscope is docked on the superior articular process (SAP)

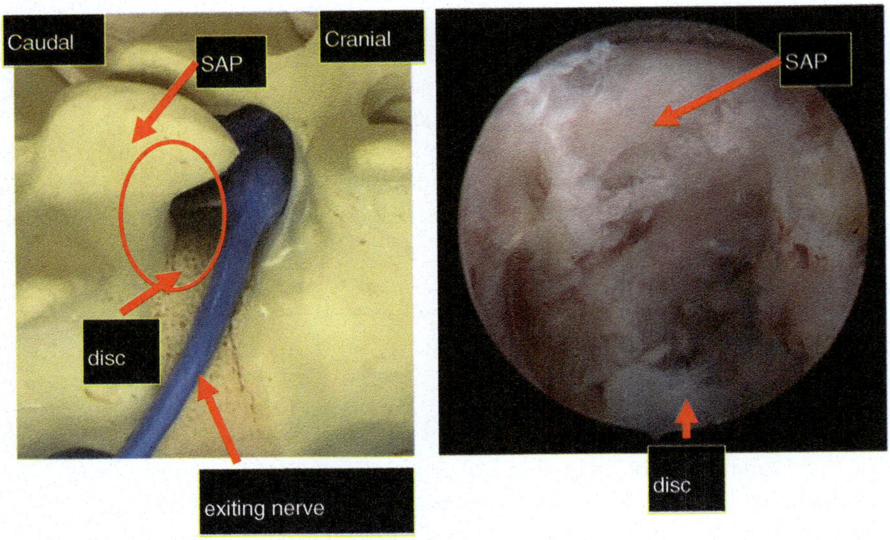

Fig. 13.4 The endoscopic view on the superior articular process (SAP). Usually, bone surface of the SAP can be seen

Fig. 13.5 KLIF starter. In case the SAP is covered with soft tissue or capsule, KLIF starter is available. The diamond particle on the surface of the KLIF starter can shave the soft tissue surrounding the SAP; then the bony surface of the SAP can be exposed

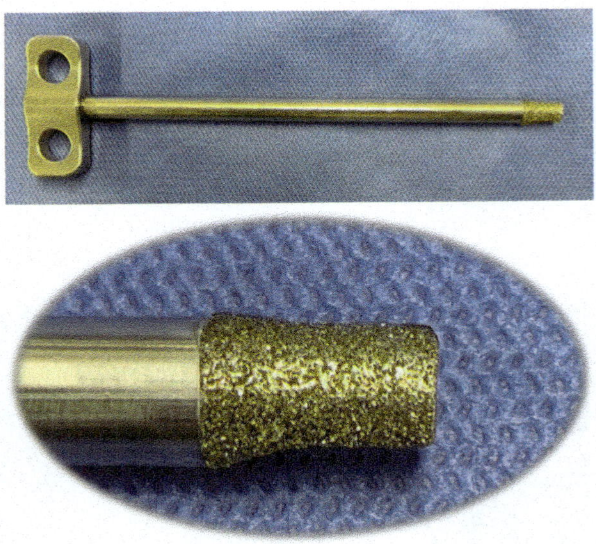

diamond particle on the surface of the KLIF starter can shave the soft tissue surrounding the SAP; then the bony surface of the SAP can be exposed.

The exposed disc distance is very important to prevent the exiting nerve root injury during the cage insertion. The width of the inserted cage is 9 mm; thus, the disc distance should be over 9 mm. As shown in Fig. 13.6, we usually create 12 mm of the disc distance (4 of 3 mm surgical drill diameter). Then, we insert a cannular with 8 mm diameter into a disc space. Through the cannula, an S-guide (K-wire

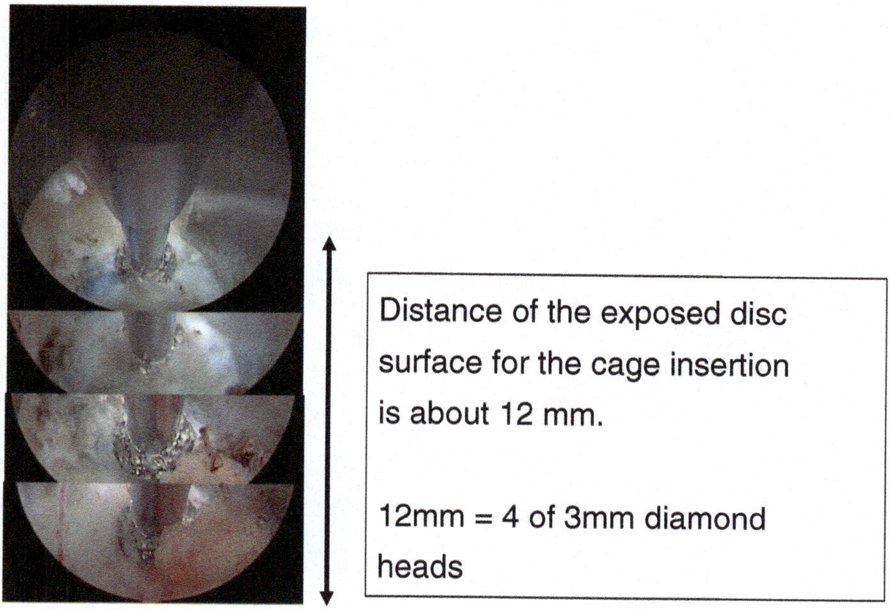

Fig. 13.6 Disc surface after full-endoscopic foraminotomy. We usually create 12 mm of the disc distance (4 of 3 mm surgical drill diameter)

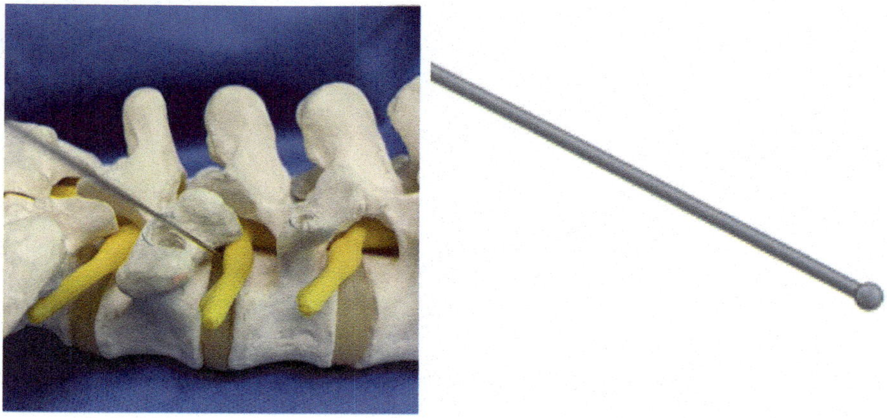

Fig. 13.7 S-guide (K-wire with a safety ball at a tip). Through the cannula, an S-guide is inserted into the disc space

with a safety ball at a tip) is inserted into the disc space (Fig. 13.7). Through the S-guide, 8–10 and 10–12 mm cannulated spacers are inserted to enlarge the disc space (Fig. 13.8). Using the spacer, the open square cannula is inserted just inside of the disc (Fig. 13.9). Through the open cannula, a specially made curette or disc shaver (Fig. 13.10) is used to empty the disc space and to curette the disc endplate (Fig. 13.11). Using the specially made bone graft funnel as shown in the left panel of Fig. 13.12, autogenic or allogenic bone is implanted. Through the open cannula,

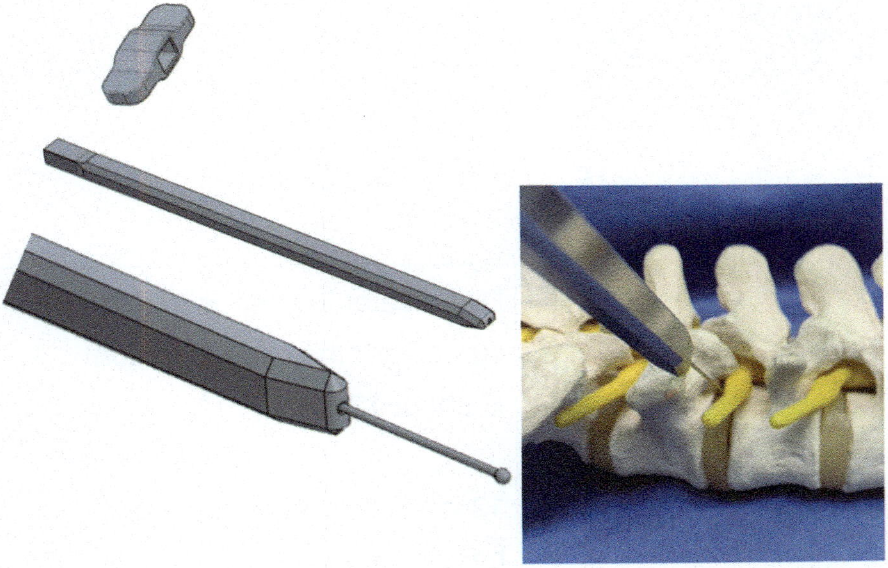

Fig. 13.8 Cannulated spacer. Through the S-guide, 8–10 and 10–12 mm cannulated spacers are inserted to enlarge the disc space

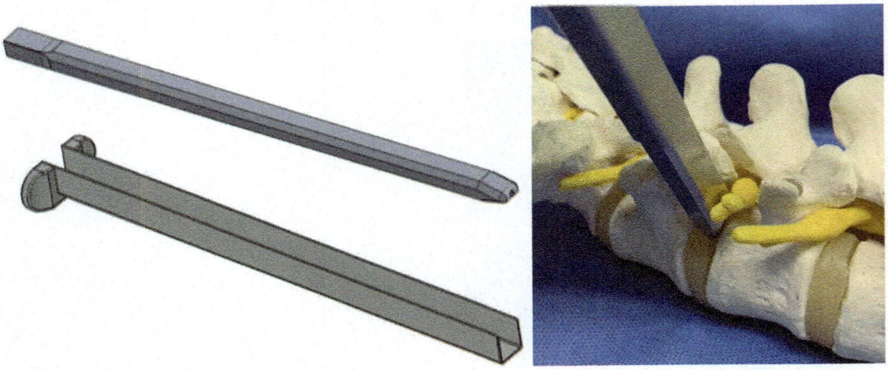

Fig. 13.9 Open square cannula. Using the spacer, the open square cannula is inserted just inside of the disc

a cubic cage is inserted as seen in the right panel of Fig. 13.12. Finally, the compression force is applied to the cage using the PPS.

Usually, indirect decompression is expected; however, if one needs direct decompression we conduct decompression surgery as the following strategy. For the central stenosis causing cauda equina syndrome, mini-open laminectomy is performed prior to the installation of the four PPS. For the foraminal and lateral recess stenosis, full-endoscopic decompression can be done after cage insertion [8–10].

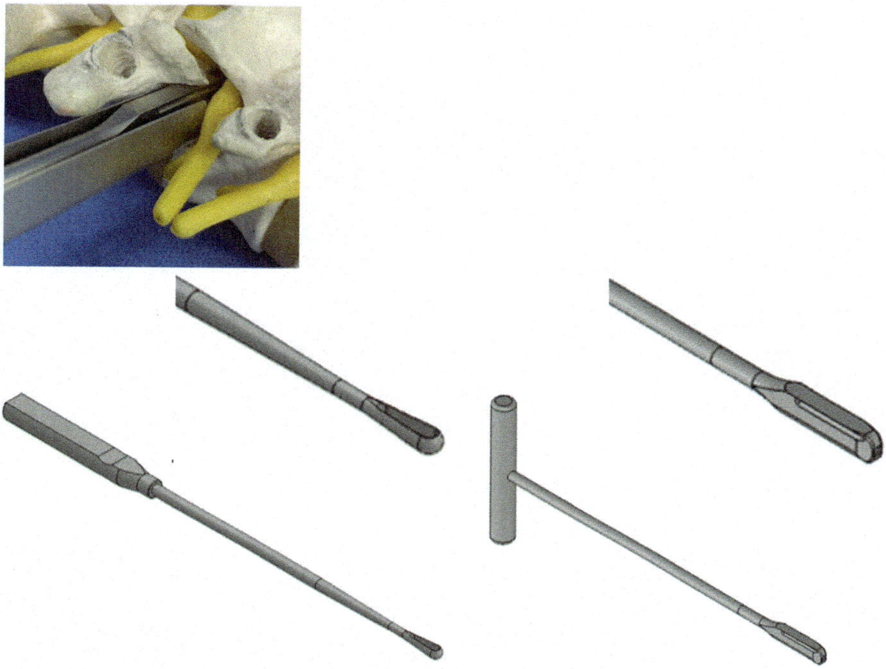

Fig. 13.10 Specially made curette and disc shaver. Through the open cannula, they are used to empty the disc space and to curette the disc endplate

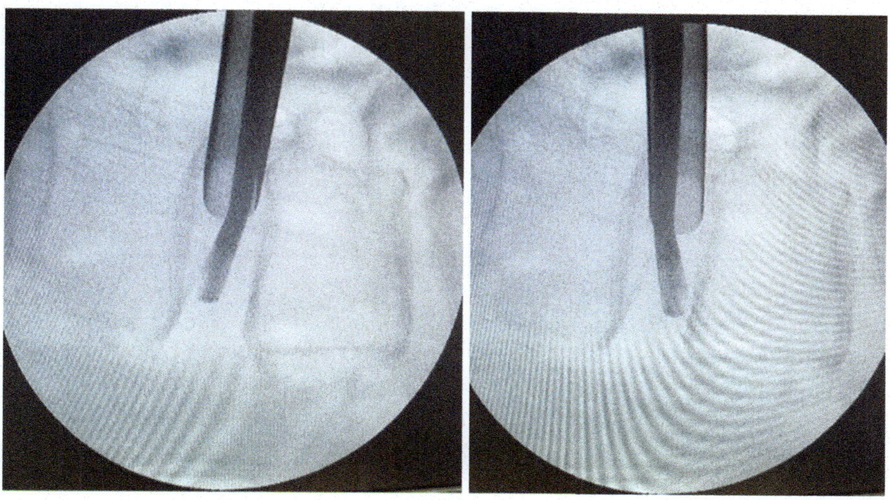

Fig. 13.11 Radiographs showing the curettage of the endoplate

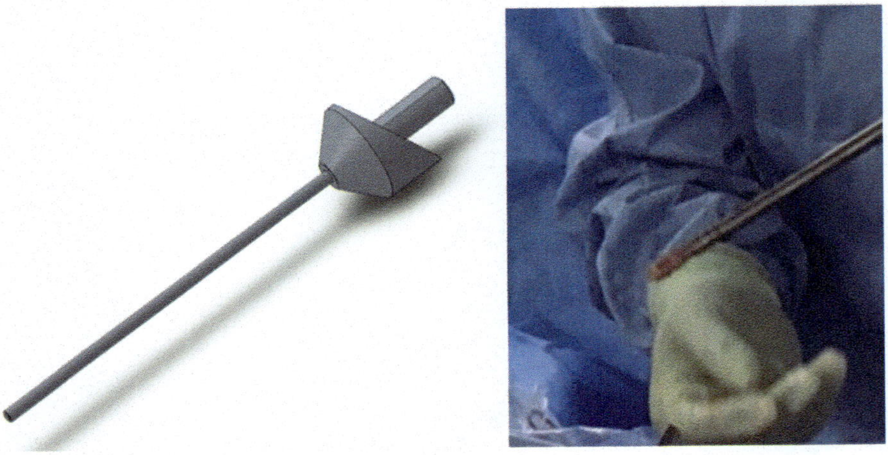

Fig. 13.12 Bone graft funnel (left) and cage insertion

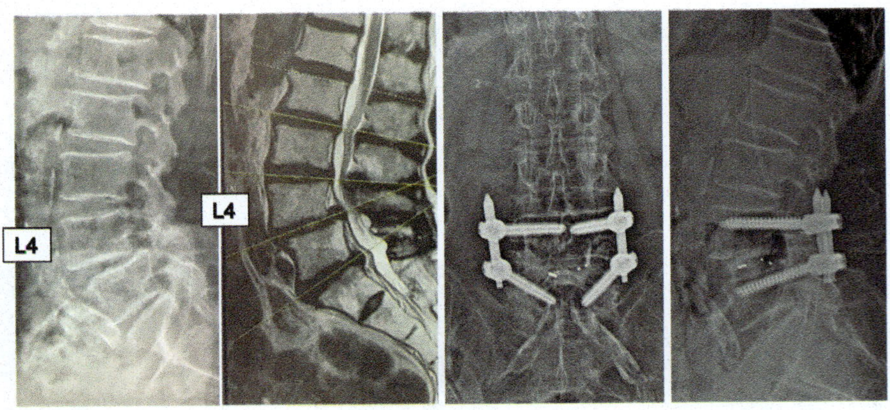

Fig. 13.13 This case is an 82 years old male

13.3 Case Presentation

We introduce a representative case in Fig. 13.13. The case is an 82 years old male. The diagnosis was L4 spondylolisthesis with lateral recess stenosis at left L4/5. He visited us complaining of low back pain and left leg pain. Previously, he had a history of laminectomy for the lumbar spinal canal stenosis at L4/5 and L5/s a long time ago. We first placed four PPSs at L4 and L5 pedicles; then, reduction of slippage was made using the PPSs. From the left side, a cannula and a full endoscope was docked on the left L4/5 facet joint, and foraminotomy was conducted until enough space for the safe cage insertion was possible. The cannula was, then, inserted into the disc space, and discectomy was conducted. A cage was inserted with allogenic bones inside. Finally, full-endoscopic ventral facetectomy was performed to decompress the L4/5 lateral recess stenosis. All through the surgery, neuro-monitoring was evaluated to avoid the exiting nerve injury. After the surgery, low back and leg pain subsided.

13.4 Conclusion

In this chapter, we explained the leading-edge technique of full-endoscopic trans-Kambin triangle interbody fusion (Fullendo-KLIF). Compared to any other LIF technique, this should be the minimally invasive technique for the cage insertion. For the cage insertion, skin incision is just 11–12 mm, and back muscle dissection would be minimum. Now, we have been conducting this surgery under general anesthesia, and it may be possible under local anesthesia.

References

1. Nakamura S, Taguchi M. Full percutaneous lumbar interbody fusion: technical note. J Neurol Surg A Cent Eur Neurosurg. 2017;78(6):601–6.
2. Youn MS, Shin JK, Goh TS, Lee JS. Full endoscopic lumbar interbody fusion (FELIF): technical note. Eur Spine J. 2018;27(8):1949–55.
3. Nagahama K, Ito M, Abe Y, Murota E, Hiratsuka S, Takahata M. Early clinical results of percutaneous endoscopic transforaminal lumbar interbody fusion: a new modified technique for treating degenerative lumbar spondylolisthesis. Spine Surg Relat Res. 2018;3(4):327–34.
4. Kamson S, Lu D, Sampson PD, Zhang Y. Full-endoscopic lumbar fusion outcomes in patients with minimal deformities: a retrospective study of data collected between 2011 and 2015. Pain Physician. 2019;22(1):75–88.
5. Tumialán LM, Madhavan K, Godzik J, Wang MY. The history of and controversy over Kambin's triangle: a historical analysis of the lumbar transforaminal corridor for endoscopic and surgical approaches. World Neurosurg. 2019;123:402–8.
6. Lewandrowski KU, Ransom NA, Ramírez León JF, Yeung A. The concept for a standalone lordotic endoscopic wedge lumbar interbody fusion: the LEW-LIF. Neurospine. 2019;16(1):82–95.
7. Sairyo K, Maeda T. Fullendo-KLIF for the anatomical nomenclature of the full-endoscope guided lumbar interbody fusion through the Kambin triangle: PELIF, PETLIF, FELIF, FE-TLIF or KLIF? EC Orthopaedics. 2019;10(9):743–5.
8. Sairyo K, Chikawa T, Nagamachi A. State-of-the-art transforaminal percutaneous endoscopic lumbar surgery under local anesthesia: discectomy, foraminoplasty, and ventral facetectomy. J Orthop Sci. 2018;23(2):229–36.
9. Sairyo K, Higashino K, Yamashita K, Hayashi F, Wada K, Sakai T, Takata Y, Tezuka F, Morimoto M, Terai T, Chikawa T, Yonezu H, Nagamachi A, Fukui Y. A new concept of transforaminal ventral facetectomy including simultaneous decompression of foraminal and lateral recess stenosis: technical considerations in a fresh cadaver model and a literature review. J Med Invest. 2017;64(1.2):1–6.
10. Sairyo K, Yamashita K, Manabe H, Ishihama Y, Sugiura K, Tezuka F, Takata Y, Sakai T, Omichi Y, Takamatsu N, Hashimoto A, Maeda T. A novel surgical concept of transforaminal full-endoscopic lumbar undercutting laminectomy (TE-LUL) for central canal stenosis of the lumbar spine with local anesthesia: a case report and literature review. J Med Invest. 2019;66(3.4):224–9.

Full-Endoscopic Debridement for Infection

14

Kosaku Higashino, Daiki Nakajima, Yugen Fujii, Keisuke Nishidono, and Koichi Sairyo

Abstract

The number of pyogenic lumbar spondylitis patients has been increasing.

The basic treatment method for pyogenic spondylitis is antibiotic therapy feeding, which predominates oral. However, many cases requiring early surgical intervention are increasing because compromised hosts in elderly patients deteriorated poor general condition and prognosis; another reason is the increase of resistant bacteria.

Minimally invasive full-endoscopic lumbar discectomy and debridement with improved endoscopic instruments and techniques can treat and change prognosis for pyogenic lumbar spondylitis.

Keywords

Pyogenic spondylitis · Minimally invasive surgery · Local anesthesia · Endoscopic surgery

14.1 Introduction

The number of pyogenic lumbar spondylitis patients has been increasing [1–3].

The reason is an increase of compromised host patients who have comorbid medical problems, such as diabetes mellitus, neoplastic diseases, leukemia, chronic

K. Higashino (✉) · Y. Fujii · K. Nishidono
Department of Orthopedics, Sikoku Medical Center for Children and Adults, Zentsuji City, Kagawa, Japan

D. Nakajima · K. Sairyo
Department of Orthopedics, Tokushima University, Tokushima, Japan

K. Sairyo (ed.), *Transforaminal Full-Endoscopic Lumbar Surgery Under the Local Anesthesia*, https://doi.org/10.1007/978-981-15-7023-0_14

renal diseases, multiple organ failures, collagen diseases, or others. Compromised host patients have a potential risk factor to induce opportunistic infection [2].

The basic treatment method for pyogenic spondylitis is antibiotic therapy feeding, which predominates oral [4]. Surgical intervention is usually reserved for cases who are unresponsive to antibiotic therapy and for patients who have developed progressive spinal deformity or instability, epidural abscesses, or neurological impairment [5].

However, many cases requiring early surgical intervention are increasing because compromised hosts in elderly patients deteriorated poor general condition and prognosis; another reason is the increase of resistant bacteria.

Conventional surgical intervention usually chooses anterior spinal fusion after conservative medical treatment such as percutaneous drainage is invalid; however there are many compromised host patients having difficulty in surgical intervention because their general condition cannot stand invasive surgery.

In compromised hosts patients with pyogenic lumbar spondylitis, minimum invasive surgery is therefore necessary. Minimally invasive full-endoscopic lumbar discectomy and debridement with improved endoscopic instruments and techniques can treat and change prognosis for pyogenic lumbar spondylitis [6–9].

14.2 Indication

The surgeon has to check the trajectory of each lumbar level using preoperative imaging because there is a diaphragm attached to the first lumbar vertebrae and whether the ribs do not interfere to approach. L5/S1 level that needs the most attention to the iliac crest high and sacral alar shape because safety triangle is very narrow space at L5/S1.

We confirm whether the patients having difficulty in keeping prone position due to general poor condition beforehand in case such as the intervertebral disc puncture to take culture inspection. Depending on the general condition, patients were examined in prone position at least 30 minutes during surgery.

14.3 Anesthesia

Local anesthesia using 1% Xylocaine combined with intravenous anesthesia was used for anesthesia. The patients should be awake during the surgery so that they can respond when the nerve roots were irritated during the procedures. An anesthesiologist added an appropriate dose of dexmedetomidine or benzodiazepine intravenously when the patient felt considerable pain during procedures. Doctors have to monitor the overall status such as respiratory status and the circulatory dynamics continuously carefully.

14.4 Surgical Procedure

The entry point to the target disc is determined under fluoroscopic guidance. Sterile preparation and draping are performed, local anesthesia is administered, a spinal needle is inserted directly into the targeted disc, and the abscess is aspirated for microorganism cultures [9].

If the approach from the presence side of the iliopsoas muscle abscess, a drainage effect is obtained. A guide wire is introduced into the targeted disc space through the spinal needle. After creating a small stab-wound incision (approximately within 1 cm), a dilator and a cannulated sleeve are guided over the wire and passed sequentially into the disc space through the safety triangle (Fig. 14.1). Fluoroscopic examination is performed under two orthogonal planes to verify the correct position of the dilator tip. The tissue dilator is then removed, and the cutting tool is inserted to harvest a biopsy specimen first. Discectomy forceps are inserted through the cannulated sleeve to extract additional tissue from the infected disc under fluoroscopic monitoring (Fig. 14.1) [6–10]. The debrided tissues typically contain necrotic disc material and parts of the vertebral endplates of adjacent vertebrae. The specimen is subjected to aerobic and anaerobic cultures, tuberculosis culture, polymerase chain

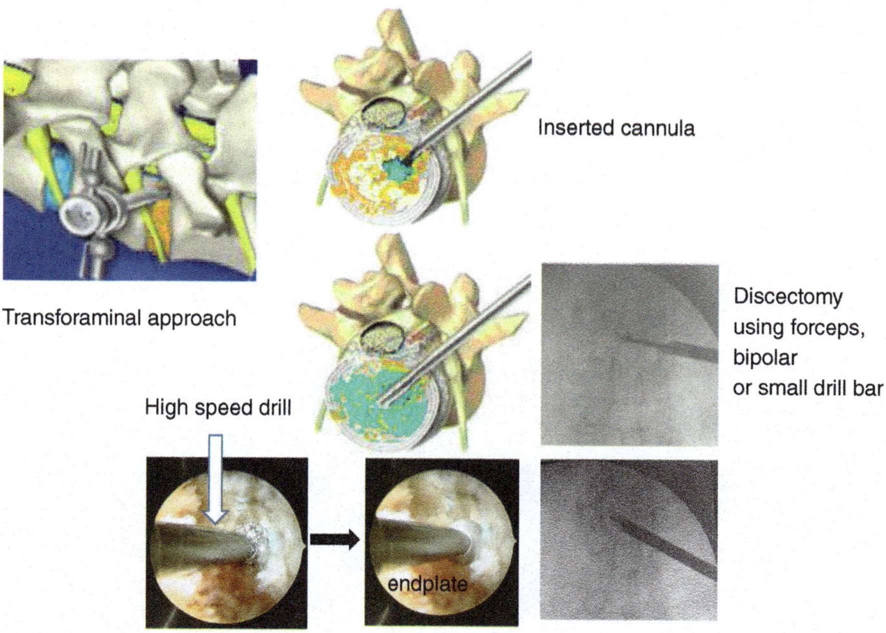

Fig. 14.1 Discectomy forceps are inserted through the cannulated sleeve to extract additional tissue from the infected disc under fluoroscopic monitoring

reaction, fungal culture, and histopathologic examinations. After biopsy and debridement, irrigation is performed using more than 2000 ml saline and the intra-discal lesion is endoscopically examined (Fig. 14.1). When the end plate was found after debridement of pulposus tissue or annulus fibrosus tissue, additional curettage may be performed a procedure using a high-speed drill. Finally, a drainage tube (diameter, 3.2 mm) is inserted into the debrided tissues.

14.5 Case Presentation

14.5.1 Case 1

60 years old-related men:

A pyogenic lumbar spondylitis and epidural abscess of L5/S1 were detected in MRI (Fig. 14.2). He underwent FED on the thirteenth day after onset.

Surgical image showed that the color of the annulus fibrosus was normal, but brown pus leaked when annulus was resected. Brown pus leaked over and over again when nucleus pulposus was resected sequentially (Fig. 14.3).

The intervertebral disc tissue still remained in the early period of infection, and a drainage effect under direct view with FED endoscope was thought to be obtained.

CRP became negative 2 months later, and the inflammatory findings improved even on an MRI, and the epidural abscess disappeared (Fig. 14.2).

14.5.2 Case 2

81 years old-related women:

She was diagnosed as having DIC due to pyelonephritis, and *Escherichia coli* was detected in blood cultures.

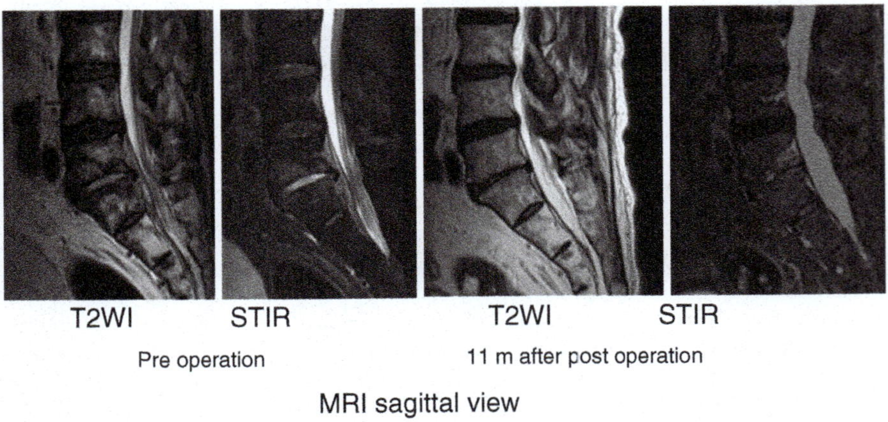

Fig. 14.2 MRI of Case 2

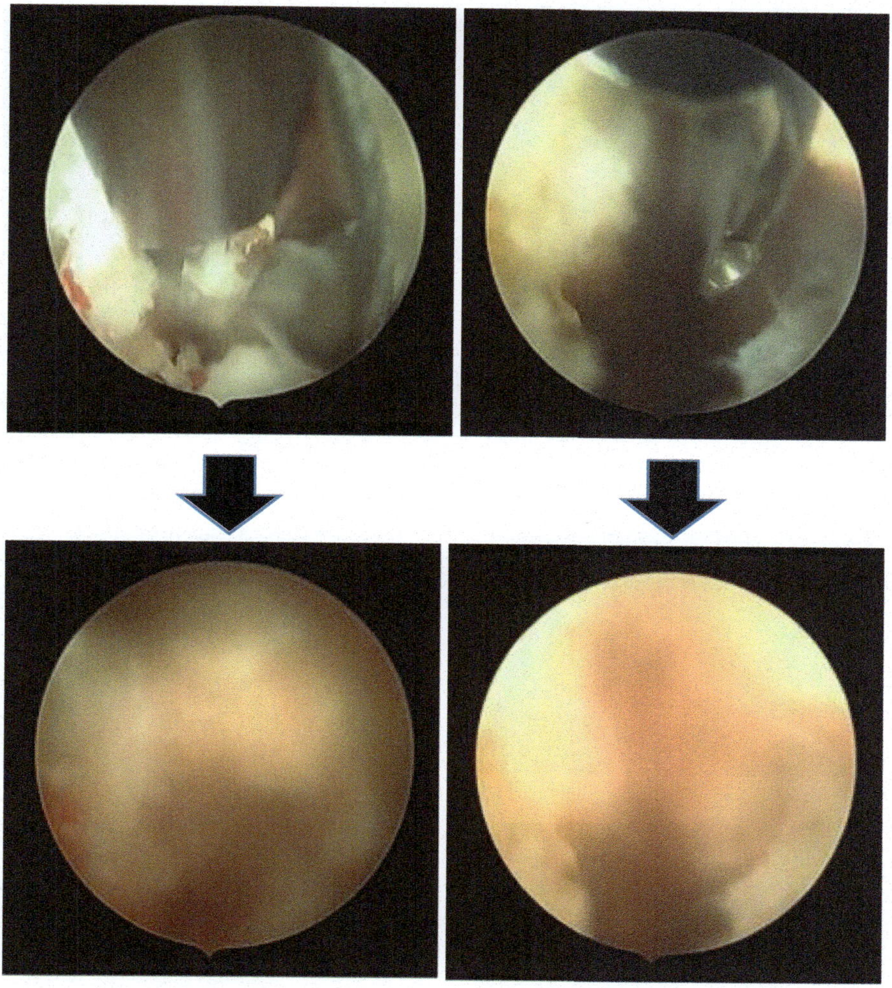

Fig. 14.3 Operative finding

MRI showed two-level pyogenic lumbar spondylitis at L3/4 and L4/5. She underwent two levels of FED 1 month after onset.

The inflammatory findings were improved and CRP became negative in 3 months after surgery.

The postoperative MRI and CT image revealed foramen stenosis due to a decrease of disc height and degenerative vertebral body (Figs. 14.4 and 14.5).

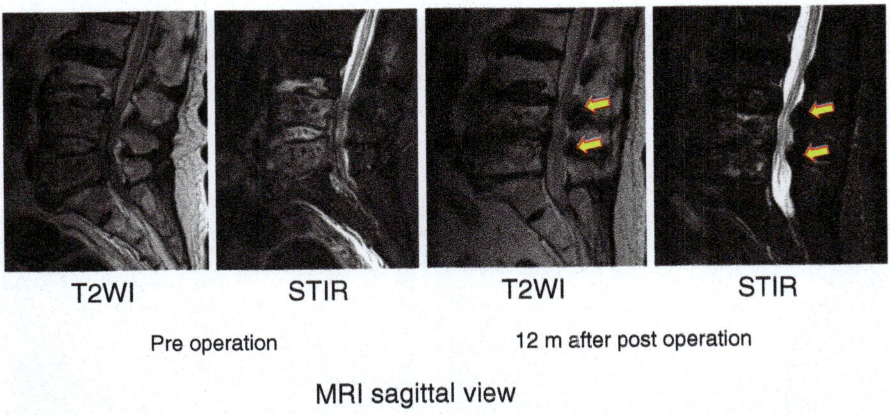

Fig. 14.4 MRI of Case 2 shows spinal canal stenosis at L3/4 and L4/5

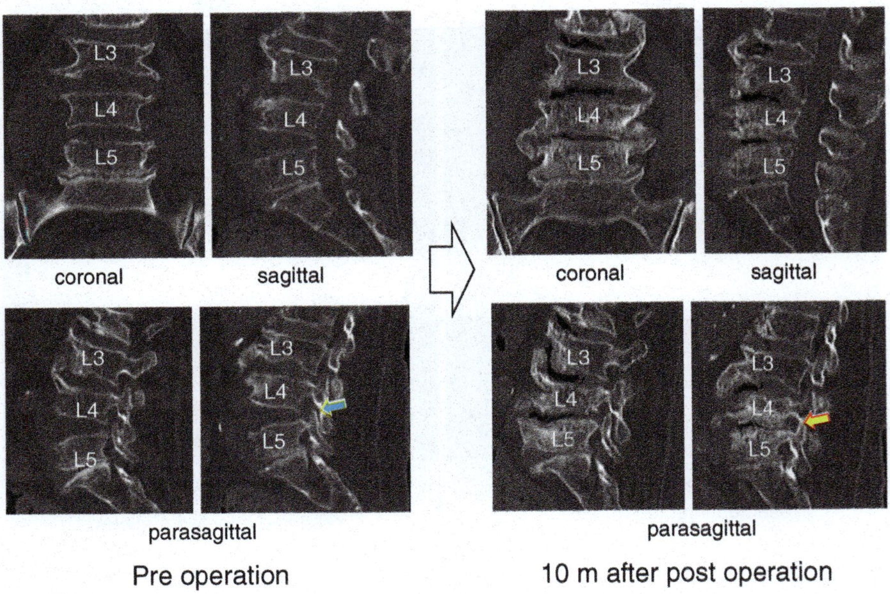

Fig. 14.5 CT of Case 2 shows the tendency for fusion between vertebral bodies, appearance of osteophyte formation, and foraminal stenosis at L3/4 and L4/5

14.6 Discussion and Conclusion

Posterolateral spinal FED debridement and irrigation resulted in satisfactory outcome for pyogenic lumbar spondylitis patients with poor general condition. Direct endoscopic observation and saline perfusion for the infected region are usually possible.

Whereas a drainage effect is limited, when an abscess enlarges in epidural space or back muscle [10]. It is suggested that it is important to choose FED treatment when conservative treatment is ineffective even with the appropriate antimicrobial agent and systemic management.

References

1. Shields D, Robinson P, Crowley TP. Iliopsoas abscess—a review and update on the literature. Int J Surg. 2012;10(9):466–9.
2. Gouliouris T, Aliyu SH, Brown NM. Spondylodiscitis: update on diagnosis and management. J Antimicrob Chemother. 2010;65(Suppl 3):iii11–24.
3. Maiuri F, Iaconetta G, Gallicchio B, Manto A, Briganti F. Spondylodiscitis. Clinical and magnetic resonance diagnosis. Spine (Phila Pa 1976). 1997;22(15):1741–6.
4. Berbari EF, Kanj SS, Kowalski TJ, Darouiche RO, Widmer AF, Schmitt SK, et al. 2015 Infectious Diseases Society of America (IDSA) clinical practice guidelines for the diagnosis and treatment of native vertebral osteomyelitis in adults. Clin Infect Dis. 2015;61(6):e26–46.
5. Rezai AR, Woo HH, Errico TJ, Cooper PR. Contemporary management of spinal osteomyelitis. Neurosurgery. 1999;44(5):1018–25; discussion 25–6.
6. Ito M, Abumi K, Kotani Y, Kadoya K, Minami A. Clinical outcome of posterolateral endoscopic surgery for pyogenic spondylodiscitis: results of 15 patients with serious comorbid conditions. Spine (Phila Pa 1976). 2007;32(2):200–6.
7. Yang SC, Chen WJ, Chen HS, Kao YH, Yu SW, Tu YK. Extended indications of percutaneous endoscopic lavage and drainage for the treatment of lumbar infectious spondylitis. Eur Spine J. 2014;23(4):846–53.
8. Yu WY, Siu C, Wing PC, Schweigel JF, Jetha N. Percutaneous suction aspiration for osteomyelitis. Report of two cases. Spine (Phila Pa 1976). 1991;16(2):198–202.
9. Fu TS, Chen LH, Chen WJ. Minimally invasive percutaneous endoscopic discectomy and drainage for infectious spondylodiscitis. Biom J. 2013;36(4):168–74.
10. Iida K, Yoshikane K, Tono O, Tarukado K, Harimaya K. The effectiveness of a percutaneous endoscopic approach in a patient with psoas and epidural abscess accompanied by pyogenic spondylitis: a case report. J Med Case Rep. 2019;13(1):253.

The manufacturer's authorised representative in the EU is Springer Nature Customer Service Centre GmbH, Europaplatz 3, 69115 Heidelberg, Germany. If you have any concerns regarding our products, please contact ProductSafety@springernature.com

Printed and bound by CPI Group (UK) Ltd, Croydon, CR0 4YY
30/09/2026
02225265-0004